Trauma Operative Procedures

Springer-Verlag Italia Srl.

G. Berlot
H. Delooz
A. Gullo (Eds)

Trauma Operative Procedures

Series edited by
Antonino Gullo

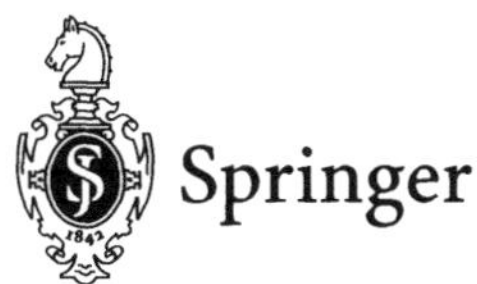

Springer

G. Berlot, MD
Department of Anaesthesia, Intensive Care and Pain Therapy
Cattinara Hospital, Trieste, Italy

H. Delooz, MD
Department of Emergency Medicine
University Hospitals, Catholic University, Leuven, Belgium

A. Gullo, MD
Department of Anaesthesia, Intensive Care and Pain Therapy
Cattinara Hospital, Trieste, Italy

Series of *Topics in Anaesthesia and Critical Care* edited by
A. Gullo, MD
Department of Anaesthesia, Intensive Care and Pain Therapy
Cattinara Hospital, Trieste, Italy

ISBN 978-88-470-0045-2   ISBN 978-88-470-2151-8 (eBook)
DOI 10.1007/978-88-470-2151-8

Library of Congress Cataloging-in-Publication Data: Applied for

Cover design: Simona Colombo, Milan
Typesetting and layout: Photolife, Milan

SPIN: 10697736

Foreword

Trauma has assumed a prominent role in contemporary medicine as an event that can significantly influence clinical variables such as morbidity, functional deficits and consequential disability, and mortality. Trauma is the principal cause of death in the population below 40 years of age in industrialized countries. Therefore, there is great interest in studying traumatic events from both the clinical and epidemiological viewpoints. The importance of trauma is exemplified by the fact that in many countries the trauma patient is first treated in specialized "trauma centers", in which the diagnostic and treatment processes are facilitated by the 24-hour presence of personnel having interdisciplinary competencies.

Trauma in this context consists of any acute, often unexpected, condition. Many of the medical difficulties associated with trauma occur in a relatively brief period that spans from the first call for help to the initiation of first aid measures. A correct approach depends on the availability of experienced personnel. The first measures of aid must guarantee, above all, the patient's survival. The most critical, initial phases of care to trauma patients are represented by the triad: first aid, triage, and transport. Specific morbidity indices, whether anatomical, functional or mixed, are indispensable elements for monitoring a patient's clinical evolution. The immediate availability of "essential" drugs is imperative to confront the clinical situations that often present in the acute post-traumatic phase.

Clinically, trauma is often synonymous with hemorrhagic shock, even if not accompanied by evident blood loss, due to internal organ lesions followed by extravasation into the retroperitoneum or splanchnic cavities. Progressive deterioration of blood circulation implies a rapid alteration in homeostasis; a significant reduction in blood flow may result in organ dysfunction or failure, leading to exitus (cerebral death) within only a few minutes.

Readiness to offer an adequate level of cure in the event of catastrophic trauma requires that: protocols describing the correct clinical approach be established according to the latest clinical research results; health workers and capable volunteers be properly trained. The general public also needs training in three fields: recognition of the urgency and of a life-threatening condition, correct alerting on the EMS system and finally first aid while waiting for the EMS. The first aid operator is characteristically manually adroit, and is able to rapidly determine and initiate the most appropriate life-saving strategy. One of the most important strategies is airway management.

In many situations in which surgery is necessary, local-regional anesthesia is indicated. The opportune establishment in many trauma centers of dedicated teams of anesthesiologists optimizes the diagnostic process and allows rapid surgical intervention.

In certain circumstances it is necessary to adopt therapeutic measures to avoid significant metabolic alterations which occur secondarily to the traumatic injury. Such measures include maintenance of body temperature to prevent hypothermia, prophylactic treatment for expected pain, and airway control to prevent or treat pulmonary inhalation of gastric fluids. Prophylactic measures are especially important in coma patients with neurological impairment subsequent to overdose. Drug use or abuse as a cause of trauma poses significant difficulties for the anaesthesiology team, both for the direct effects of such substances on the patient and in consideration of the drugs' possible interactions with anesthetics.

It is recommended to update the guidelines regarding the indications for blood transfusion and fluid therapy to sustain adequate circulation. Also useful are guidelines describing strategies to avoid alterations in haematologic and renal homeostasis. Particular attention must be directed to monitoring the trauma patient in the immediate post-operative period and to evaluating when to proceed with intensive care treatment. A thorough overview of the clinical issues inherent to trauma must take into consideration medical guidelines for both basic life support (BLS) and advanced life support.

November 1998

Antonino Gullo, MD

Contents

Contributors

Agrò F.
Department of Anaesthesiology and Intensive Care, University School of Medicine, Campus Bio-Medico, Roma, Italy.

Baron J.F.
Department of Anaesthesiology and Intensive Care, Broussais Hospital, Paris, France.

Baskett J.F.
Department of Anaesthesia, Frenchay Hospital, Bristol, UK.

Berlot G.
Department of Anesthesia and Intensive Care, University of Trieste, Cattinara Hospital, Italy.

Boldt J.
Department of Anesthesiology and Intensive Care Medicine, Klinikum der Stadt Ludwigshafen, Germany.

Bronselaer K.
Department of Emergency Medicine, University Hospitals Leuven, Belgium.

Cerchiari E.
S.S.U.Em 118, I° Department of Anaesthesiology and Intensive Care Medicine, Niguarda Hospital, Milan, Italy.

Crawford M.E.
Department of Anaesthesiology, Bispebjerg University Hospital, Copenhagen, Denmark.

Delooz H.
Department of Emergency Medicine, University Hospitals, Catholic University, Leuven, Belgium.

Desjardins G.
Ryder Trauma Centre, University of Miami, Florida, USA.

Di Filippo A.
Institute of Anaesthesiology and Intensive Care, University of Florence, Florence, Italy.

Dick W.F.
Klinik für Anästhesiologie, Johannes Gutenberg-Universität Mainz, Mainz, Germany.

Gillis M.
Department of Emergency Medicine, Hospitals of Lier, Belgium.

Grauer M.T.
Department of Neurology, University of the Saarland, Homburg/Saar, Germany.

Gullo A.
Department of Anesthesia and Intensive Care, University of Trieste, Cattinara Hospital, Italy.

Hadfield R.J.H.
Liverpool Hospital, University of New South Wales, Sydney, Australia.

Inghilleri G.
Department of Immunohaemathology, Gaetano Pini Hospital, Milano, Italy.

Lingnau W.
Department of Anaesthesia and Intensive Care Medicine, Leopold-Franzens-University, Innsbruck, Austria.

Lipp M.
Klinik für Anästhesiologie, Johannes Gutenberg-Universität Mainz, Mainz, Germany.

Mercuriali F.
Department of Immunohaemathology, Gaetano Pini Hospital, Milano, Italy.

Nolan J.P.
Royal United Hospital, Bath, UK.

Novelli G.P.
Institute of Anaesthesiology and Intensive Care, University of Florence, Florence, Italy.

Parr M.J.A.
Liverpool Hospital, University of New South Wales, Sydney, Australia.

Rask H.
Department of Anaesthesiology, Bispebjerg University Hospital, Copenhagen, Denmark.

Sesana G.
S.S.U.Em 118, I° Department of Anaesthesiology and Intensive Care Medicine, Niguarda Hospital, Milan, Italy.

Sutcliffe A.J.
Department of Anaesthesia and Intensive Care, Queen Elizabeth Hospital, Edgbaston, Birmingham, England.

Treib J.
Department of Neurology, University of the Saarland, Homburg/Saar, Germany.

Trillò G.
Department of Anesthesia and Intensive Care, University of Trieste, Cattinara Hospital, Italy.

van Camp L.A.
Ministry of the Flemish Community, Administration of Health Care, Belgium.

Chapter 1

Planning, organisation, education, triage and research in immediate medical care: an introduction

J.F. BASKETT

Immediate medical care may mean different things to different people. For the purposes of this chapter, immediate medical care shall be considered as extending from the time of injury or onset of acute illness until such time as the patient is delivered to specialist definitive care. This period covers the prehospital phase and the reception and initial management of the patient in the admitting area or emergency room of the hospital.

Planning and organisation

In planning and organising an immediate medical care service, certain fundamental factors should be considered. These may be influenced by previous national or local practice and tradition but these features alone should not dictate the implementation of an optimal service. Key factors will include:
1. public education;
2. a system to provide access to the service;
3. local infrastructure geography and size of area served;
4. road and air services potential;
5. communications;
6. support services;
7. personnel available to provide prehospital and hospital emergency room care;
8. specialist hospital services available;
9. finance available.

Public education

The results achieved by the professionals will be enormously enhanced by the trained and educated bystander who is able to provide simple airway control, artificial ventilation, control of overt peripheral haemorrhage and basic life support using cardiopulmonary resuscitation (CPR). Most striking results occur with bystander CPR buying time until defibrillation is available but many other victims are saved from "second injury" by simple airway control in the head injured, drowning or poisoned patient. Patients have been spared from exsanguination by simple wound compression when major accessible blood vessels have been severed. Fatal hypothermia has been prevented by intelligent prophylaxis by first aiders.

Access to the emergency medical system (EMS)

Bystander assistance in the seriously ill or injured is futile, however, unless there is a system for rapid access to the professional service. A dedicated emergency phone number should allow immediate access to the major emergency services including police, fire and the emergency immediate medical care service. In the UK the 999 service has been available for 62 years; the US and Canada have developed a 911 system over the past 30-40 years. Single emergency access telephone numbers are still not completely developed in all European countries. With cross boundary flow increasing annually, it is time for the pan European universal emergency telephone number (112) to be introduced throughout the region.

Local infrastructure, geography and size of area served

The nature of the service required will be dictated by the local geography and size of area served. Urban areas generally enjoy easy access for land ambulances but suffer from a high incidence of inner city violence, industrial and transport accidents. Inner city violence is associated with a high incidence of penetrating trauma and drug related illness which may put healthcare personnel at risk. Fires in densely populated areas such as high rise apartments may overwhelm the local burn specialty facility.

Local features such as mountains and water hazards (lakes, rivers and coastlines) will require specialist training and competence from the service. In many countries a partnership with military personnel operating a search and rescue (SAR) service has been established to amplify and support the local immediate medical care service.

If the area served is extensive and rural, response and transit times will, perforce, be prolonged. This will throw extra dependence on the bystander and will require extra skills from the professionals. The emphasis when transit times are long moves away from a policy of rapid removal of the patient to hospital and veers towards a policy of stabilisation prior to transport, even though some time is required to achieve this.

Road and air services potential

There is little doubt that helicopter (or even fixed wing aircraft) offer the best option for rapid transfer to specialist medical facilities in extremely rural areas where land access may be difficult or roads congested. Helicopter transport, however, is not without danger and is limited by night flying or bad weather. Access is limited in urban areas for safe helicopter landing. In urban areas, road transport is usually favoured. Response times are quicker and easy access is usually possible. Nonetheless, some centres, i.e., Royal London Hospital Helicopter Emergency Medical System (HEMS) have developed a successful service operating from the hospital to serve a large congested conurbation and similar systems operate, for example, in cities in France, Germany, Switzerland, Austria and the United States and Canada. However, there is little doubt that the helicopter comes into its own in rural areas where land access is difficult or protracted such as in the fjords of Scandinavia or the mountains of the Alpine countries.

Communications

Aside from public access to the service good communications are essential with the service and between the service and local and specialist hospitals. The majority of systems rely upon radio but satellite telephones, telemetry and visual links offer enormous potential improvements for advice. Transponders provide transfer of information data immediate location of vehicles at any moment in time and offer tremendous improvement in efficiency of resource deployment.

Support services

No immediate medical care service can operate in isolation without the support of the police, fire service and specialist units such as chemical incident groups, life boats and SAR services. The support of these allied services is particularly essential in the major incident with multiple casualties and specific hazards.

Personnel available

There is considerable variation between country to country in the origin and nature of personnel providing an immediate medical care service in the prehospital arena. The choice of personnel is dictated by tradition, finance and availability. It is now generally agreed that considerable skills and expertise are required for effective prehospital care and that a cadre of professionals, who are well trained and expert at all aspects of advanced trauma and cardiac life support, is essential to any system responding to the seriously ill and injured. Some countries have chosen to train the non-physician paramedic for this role, others have focused on specially trained nurses and yet others have provided doctors (generally anaesthesiologists but occasionally cardiologists and trauma surgeons). Those services using doctors generally operate a two tier system, while many paramedic based services operate a single tier system, dependent on the information received from the caller. Further research is required to evaluate whether the extra potential benefit accruing from physician response justifies the extra expense and the need to train considerably more doctors. What is very clear, however, is that paramedic – and nurse – based systems must be subject to education, training and control by physicians concerned with emergency care. Without this involvement the service stagnates and will not progress safely. Innovations in prehospital care can only be introduced after they have been subjected to scientific medical scrutiny and the physicians involved must also be aware of the limitations of skills placed upon the prehospital personnel and the environment they work in.

There is no doubt that standards within a country should be uniform and a national training formula should be created with a national audit to ensure a uniform high standard of performance. Hopefully and possibly such standards should transgress boundaries within Europe so that at least a basic level of care can be expected through the continent regardless of the detailed design and organisation of the individual systems.

Within the hospital the specialty of Emergency Medicine has developed and become established in the UK, Australia, Canada and the USA and other former British colonies. However, the specialty, with a few notable exceptions, has not become established in continental Europe where management by the traditional specialties of anaesthesia, medicine and surgery hold sway as appropriate. Those with experience of working with the specialty of Emergency Medicine are able to recognise its virtues as it provides clinical expertise in breadth across traditional specialist boundaries and makes for an altogether more efficient EMS. The specialty will fail, however, if it attempts to work in isolation from the specialist disciplines and the best services work in harmony with anaesthesia, surgery and radiology in the field of trauma and with anaesthesia and cardiology and internal medicine in medical emergencies. The emergency physician has a co-ordinating role in serious and life threatening emergencies and ensures that no stone is left unturned in the overall management of the patient – a situation which may arise if the patient is allocated to a single specialist who may be blind to an illness or injury outside their own sphere of expertise or interest.

Specialist hospital services available

The immediate medical care service should be designed around the available hospital services. In an urban area the patient should be taken to the nearest appropriate hospital for that patient's illness or injury. This may mean by-passing the nearest hospital. In rural areas with potentially long transit times, it may be wise to take the patient first to the nearest hospital for stabilisation along ATLS or ACLS principles prior to secondary transfer for specialist definitive care.

Protocols should be established for such decisions which will depend on the expertise of the prehospital personnel, the transport arrangements and the facilities and expertise at the local hospital.

Finance

The service which is to be established will depend on the finances available. The best investment is in the training of the personnel in the service and a concentration on the commonest conditions with a view to providing the greatest good for the greatest number.

Education

The hallmark of immediate medical care education centres around the principles of ATLS, ACLS and APLS. For sure, these elements of training are essential for the seriously ill and injured as seen through the eyes of the hospital based specialist but the spectrum of work encountered in the EMS extends over and above the core material of these programmes. Modifications to emphasise the prehospital priorities are included in the PHTLS course of the Royal College of Surgeons and the Diploma in Immediate Medical Care (Dip. Imm. Med. Care) and the Prehospital Emergency Care Course of the Royal College of Surgeons of Edinburgh and British Association for Immediate Care. Similar courses are run in France and Germany. In Europe, courses in Disaster Medicine are run at CEMEC in Italy and by the British Association for Immediate Care at Cambridge. Such courses emphasise not only the ATLS, ACLS and APLS doctrine but extend further to include splinting, entrapment and extrication in the field, triage, communication skills, etc. Paramedic training in the UK conforms to a national standard formulated by the National Health Service Training Directive advised by medical representatives of all the specialist Royal Colleges. Paramedics are trained at regional training centres and local hospitals all of which must conform to national training standards using national training manuals and protocols. Their training is supervised by Local Paramedic Training Committees composed of doctors drawn from all relevant specialties. Maintenance of paramedic status is dependent on regular refresher training.

Emergency medical technicians have also national standards to achieve and their sphere of expertise includes basic trauma and cardiac life support, automated defibrillation, airway control using the laryngeal mask, and glucagon and salbutamol administration. All must pass through the emergency medical technician ranks before progressing to paramedic training.

Triage is required when there is more than one patient and is especially important in major incidents with multiple casualties.

The overriding principle is to do the greatest good for the greatest number and this may involve department from the protocols relating to a single patient.

A rapid assessment of all accessible patients by the most experienced member of the team is a vital first step. Ideally this leader should be accompanied by assistants who can be asked to deal simply and immediately with life threatening conditions such as the obstructed airway or control of haemorrhage from peripheral sources. Once these situations have been addressed then the leader can begin to allocate triage and treatment priorities to individual patients. In principle the first to be evacuated to hospital should be the most seriously ill or injured but those with injuries who are unlikely to survive should give way to those with a good chance of recovery.

Although the seriously injured should have priority, it may be that, in fact, the "walking" wounded arrive at hospital first, either because they have used independent transport (own car, bus, etc.) or because on site treatment may impose a delay in evacuating the seriously ill.

Local pre-event major incident planning between all the rescue and medical services is an essential element of success and certain principles should be adhered to. It is unwise to draw the field medical team from the designated receiving hospitals; it is better to train a special team(s) from another centre and retain staff at the receiving hospitals. It is also wise to designate more than one receiving hospital in a given area so that disruption to normal work is minimised.

Research

Research opportunities abound in Emergency Medicine and the service it provides. By and large the fields of research can be grouped into: 1) biomedical; 2) clinical; 3) organisation.

Biomedical

In this area further work is needed into the biomechanics of injuries and the effects of injury at both organ and cellular level particularly in head trauma and the burned patient. The fields of study extend from forensic analysis of the site and the source of injury to laboratory studies in vivo and in vitro.

Clinical

In the clinical field the value of prehospital thrombolysis in both cardiac and stroke patients requires study and evaluation. The application of permissive hypotension in penetrating trauma requires investigation outside the urban environment and its relevance in blunt trauma requires study in both the urban and rural scene.

In CPR the ventilation required in the cardiac arrested patient needs to be studied in the light of the need for oxygenation and carbon dioxide removal versus the benefit of an adequate and possibly increased number of chest compressions achieved in the minute.

The study of outcome pioneered by the Major Trauma Outcome Study (MTOS) needs continuing audit on a multinational scale and such studies need to be applied to other emergency conditions. Further refinement of scoring systems in trauma and other conditions is required and a template for reporting traumatic injuries is being designed on a similar basis to the Utstein system for reporting cases of cardiac arrest.

Organisation

A study of criteria based dispatch of the service is required on a national and European scale. More precise definitions of the indications for helicopter transport vs land ambulance are needed together with the pros and cons of each method in specific environments.

Further research is needed into the potentials of telemetry including visual transfer so that the receiving hospital are not only made aware of the vital signs but may also conduct a visual examination of the patient.

Above all results achieved by the service must be audited so that valuable activities may be justified, highlighted and supported financially, and systems and interventions which are not shown to be useful may be deleted.

Further readings

1. Grande CM (1993) Text book of trauma anaesthesia and critical care. Mosby Year Book, St Louis
2. Westaby S (1989) Trauma pathogenesis and treatment. Heinemann, Oxford
3. Baskett PJF, Weller RM (1988) Medicine for disasters. Wright/Butterworth, London
4. Greaves I, Hodgetts T, Porter K (1995) Handbook for immediate care. WB Saunders, London
5. Baskett PJF (1993) Resuscitation handbook, 2nd Ed, Mosby, London
6. Baskett PJF, Dow AAC, Nolan JP, Maull K (1995) Practical procedures in anaesthesia and critical care. Mosby, London
7. Howarth PA, Evans RJ (1994) Key Topics in accident and emergency medicine. Bios, Oxford
8. Robertson C, Redmond AD (1991) The management of major trauma. Oxford University, Oxford
9. Murray V (1990) Major chemical disasters - medical aspects of management. Royal Society of Medicine Services, London
10. Colquohoun MC, Handley AJ, Evans TR (1998) ABC of resuscitation, 4th ed. BMJ, London
11. ABC of major trauma (1966) 2nd ed. BMJ, London
12. Bossaert L (1998) Guidelines for resuscitation. The European Resuscitation Council. Elsevier, Amsterdam

Chapter 2

Current trauma scoring systems and their applications: a review

L.A. Van Camp, H. Delooz

Trauma is the consequence of an external cause of injury that results in tissue damage or destruction produced by intentional or unintentional exposure to thermal, mechanical, electrical, or chemical energy, or by the absence of heat or oxygen.

"Injury is a threat to health in every country in the world and is currently responsible for 7% of world mortality" [1]. In the US, as in most industrialized societies, trauma is the leading cause of death from childhood to the fourth decade of live. Injuries, fatal and non-fatal, result in an important financial and productivity loss while inflicting a tremendous personal burden on the injured and their families [2]. This universal problem needs a worldwide approach.

The principal goal of this approach, known as "Injury Control", is to reduce injury mortality, morbidity and disability. This goal can only be reached through implementation of prevention strategies, based on recent injury epidemiology and through continuous assesment and improvement of the quality of trauma care.

Trauma scoring mechanisms serve a threesome purpose. First of all, they are used for triage, secondly they become an essential tool in trauma care management, where they have been applied in patient outcome evaluation, quality assessment and resource allocation, and thirdly they are fundamental in trauma epidemiology.

Many trauma scores and scales have been developed during the last 30 years. Table 1 gives a comprehensive summary of these scales.

This article focuses only on the most universally applied trauma scoring and scaling systems and discusses how they can be applied in injury control.

Types of trauma scoring systems

Physiological trauma scoring systems

Injury can cause physiological changes in a victim's body. These physiological changes are reflected by changes in vital signs and level of consciousness, which are normally assessed as part of the first survey. Physiological trauma scoring systems are based on the measurement of vital signs and/or level of consciousness. Such scales are commonly used for patient triage and for assessing response to therapy. Combined with anatomical scores, physiological scores can also be used for prediction of patient's outcome, comparison of trauma populations and quality assurance.

Table 1. Summary of existing trauma scoring systems

Name	Abbreviation	Reference
SIMBOL Rating and Evaluation System	SIMBOL	[46]
Trauma Index		[47]
Abbreviated Injury Scale	AIS	[16]
		[28, 17]
Comprehensive Injury Scale	CRIS	[48]
Prognostic Index for Severe Trauma		[49]
Glasgow Coma Scale	GCS	[3]
Renal Index		[51]
Therapeutic Intervention Scoring System	TISS	[52]
		[53]
Injury Severity Score	ISS	[19]
		[20]
		[21]
Respiratoy Index	RI	[56]
CHOP Index		[55]
Illness-Injury Severity Index	IISI	[54]
Clinical Assessment Research and Education	CARE	[57]
Triage Index		[4]
Modified Injury Severity Scale	MISS	[58]
		[59]
Anatomic Index	AI	[60]
Hospital Trauma Index		[61]
Shock Score		[5]
Acute Physiology and Chronic Health Evaluation	APACHE	[62]
Trauma Score	TS	[5]
Penetrating Abdominal Trauma Index		[63]
Probability of Death Score	PODS	[64]
Circulation Respiration Abdomen Motor Speech Scale	CRAMS	[65]
Preliminary Method	PRE	[39]
State Transition Screen	STS	[39]
Definitive Methodology	DEF	[39]
Mangled Extremity Syndrome	MES	[66]
Acute Physiology and Chronic Health Evaluation II	APACHE II	[67]
Prehospital Index		[68]
Revised Trauma Score	RTS	[8]
Acute Physiology and Chronic Health Evaluation III	APACHE III	[69]
Trauma Score - Injury Severity Score	TRISS	[35]
Pediatric Trauma Score	PTS	[70]
Outcome Predictive Score	OPS	[71]
Riya & Intensive Care Programme	RIP	[72]
Organ Injury Scaling	OIS	[73]
Anatomic Profile	AP	[25]
A Severity Characterization of Trauma	ASCOT	[36]
Injury Impairment Scale	IIS	[29]

The best physiological trauma severity scoring systems are based on a limited number of valid parameters that are easy to measure (by doctors, nurses and paramedics), with a high intra- and interobserver reliability and have a good predictive power (correlate well with mortality).

The state-of-the-art physiological trauma scoring system currently used is the Revised Trauma Score (RTS), in which the Glasgow Coma Scale (GCS) is incorporated.

The Glasgow Coma Scale

The Glasgow Coma Scale (GCS) was developed in 1974 by Jennett and Teasdale [3]. It became the most widely used system of defining the level of consciousness of patients with craniocerebral injuries because of its simplicity, its predictive power and its good interobserver reliability. The GCS defines the level of consciousness according to three parameters: eye-opening, best verbal response and best motor response. These parameters are comprised of three different subscales which in turn consist of a hierarchy of responses that are assigned numerical values (Table 2). The score for each subscale is determined by stimulating the patient and observing the best response. Ranging from 3 to 15, the GCS score is the sum of the scores for eye-opening, best verbal and motor response.

As this scale can assess brain function, brain damage and patient progress in consciousness, it correlates with survival and morbidity and is known as a reliable predictive measure, especially in neurotrauma [3]. The GCS not only helps to predict outcome but also serves as a guide in triage and initial patient management.

Table 2. Glasgow Coma Scale

Parameter	Response	Score
Eye-opening	Spontaneous	4
	To voice	3
	To pain	2
	None	1
Verbal response	Oriented	5
	Confused	4
	Inappropriate words	3
	Incomprehensible sounds	2
	None	1
Motor response	Obeys cornmands	6
	Localizes pain	5
	Withdraw (pain)	4
	Flexion (pain)	3
	Extension (pain)	2
	None	1

The Revised Trauma Score

In 1980 Champion et al. [4] developed the Triage Index, using pattern recognition and mathematical and statistical techniques on nearly 60 biochemical and physiological variables that were known to correlate with mortality following blunt trauma.

Weighted values of the five most important variables (eye-opening, verbal response, motor response, respiratory expansion and capillary refill) were taken to create this index. The Triage Index was the first index that could really predict patient outcome.

One year after its development, the Triage Index was modified by addition of respiratory rate and systolic blood pressure to create the Trauma Score (TS) (Table 3) [5]. This score ranges from 1 (worst) to 16 (normal). It correlates with mortality better than the Triage Index did [6], and was found to be as accurate for penetrating trauma as for blunt trauma [7].

Table 3. Trauma Score

Parameter	Value	Score
RR (per minute)	10-24	4
	25-35	3
	>35	2
	0-10	1
	0	0
RE	normal	1
	retractive	0
SBP (mmHg)	>90	4
	71-90	3
	51-70	2
	1-50	1
	0	0
CR	<2 sec	2
	>2sec	1
	no CR	0
GCS	14-15	5
	11-13	4
	8-10	3
	5-7	2
	3-4	1

RR, respiratory rate; *RE,* respiratory effort; *SBP,* systolic blood pressure; *CR,* capillary refill; *GCS,* Glasgow Coma Scale

The Revised Trauma Score (RTS) [8] was developed to be simpler than its predecessor, (i.e. respiratory expansion and capillary refill were no longer included as variables). Field use of the Trauma Score revealed that these variables were difficult to assess at night, and that the observation of "retractive" respiratory expansion had a very poor intra- and interobserver reliability. Further, there was concern that the Trauma Score underestimated the severity of some types of head injuries [8].

Currently, the RTS is the best and most universally used physiological trauma severity scoring system. Use of the RTS coded values in the field can allow rapid characterization of neurologic, circulatory, and respiratory distress and assessment of the severity of serious head injuries [8]. The predictive value of a RTS with any value below normal (positive test) to fatality, reported by Champion et al. was 96.9%. This is better than the positive predictive values (76%-92%) reported for the TS [9-11]. However, several studies have criticized the RTS as a triage tool [12, 13]. This will be discussed later.

The coded RTS values are not just tools for triage and evaluation of a patient's progress. Appropriately weighted and in combination with quantified information about the anatomical injuries, the RTS values also play an important role in outcome evaluation and quality assessment. For this type of application the coded values of GCS, systolic blood pressure, and respiratory rate are weighted and summed to yield the TRTS which takes values from 0 (worst prognosis) to 7.84 (best prognosis) (Table 4).

Table 4. Revised Trauma Score

Parameter	Value	Score
RR (per minute)	10-29	4
	>29	3
	6-9	2
	1-5	1
	0	0
SBP (mmHg)	>89	4
	76-89	3
	50-75	2
	1-49	1
	0	0
GCS	13-15	4
	9-12	3
	6-8	2
	4-5	1
	3	0

RTS, 0.9368 (GCS value) + 0.7326 (SBP value) + 0.2908 (RR value)/*RR*, respiratory rate; *SBP*, systolic blood pressure; *GCS*, Glasgow Coma Scale

Anatomical trauma scoring systems

A good anatomical scoring system must be based on a complete description of anatomical injuries, obtained from clinical evaluation, radiology, surgery, and/or autopsy. Post-mortem examination is particularly important because it often reveals previously undetected injuries [14, 15].

Where physiological scores are assigned at first contact and repeated to oversee a patient's progress, anatomical scores are usually assigned after complete diagnosis (often at discharge or post mortem). This makes them less useful as triage tools or for the assessment of response to therapy. They are mainly used to classify injured patients and/or to quantiiFy injury severity. A score that can classify and quantify injury according to severity (threat to life) can be used for prediction of outcome.

Abbreviated Injury Scale

The Abbreviated Injury Scale (AIS) [17] is an expertise and consensus derived, anatomically based system that classifies more than 2000 individual injuries by body region on a 6-point ordinal severity (threat to life) scale ranging from AIS 1 (minor) to AIS 6 (currently untreatable). The nine AIS body regions are: *1* head, *2* face, *3* neck, *4* thorax, *5* abdomen, *6* spine, *7* upper extremities, *8* lower extremities, *9* external.

The AIS is not an interval scale, i.e. the increase in injury severity from AIS 1 to 2 is much less than the increase from AIS 3 to 4, or 4 to 5.

Regular revision of the AIS is necessary because using the scale draws attention to over- or underestimation of the severity of some injuries. Also, the prognosis of trauma changes with the progress of trauma care. The AIS90 [17] is the most recent and currently most used system for scaling the severity of anatomical injury.

The main limitations of the AIS are that the scale does not assess the combined effects of multiple injuries in one patient, that it is not an interval scale and that for some (secondary) injuries severity scaling is dynamic and can be affected by the time of diagnosis (i.e., as the volume of a intracerebral hematoma can change over time, the AIS score assigned will depend on the moment that such a hematoma is documented).

Recently, software (ICDMAP-90) that converts International Classification of Deseases 9th revision Clinical Modification (ICD-9-CM) codes into AIS90 has been developed [18]. As the mapping between ICD-9-CM and AIS is not always a one-to -one correspondence, it should be emphasized that the use of the ICDMAP-90 does not replace careful AIS coding. It was developed principally for application to large, pre-existing databases where AIS scoring directly from medical records is not an option [18].

Injury Severity Score

The Injury Severity Score (ISS) [19-21] is an ordinal ascending summary severity score ranging from 0 (no injury) to 75 (severely injured) that takes into account the effect of multiple injuries in one patient. Any patient with an AIS 6 injury is assigned an ISS of 75. Otherwise the ISS is the sum of squares of the highest AIS code in each of the three most severely injured ISS body regions. The six body regions of injuries used in the ISS are: *1* head and neck, *2* face, *3* thorax, *4* abdomen, *5* extremities, *6* external.

Although this score is purely empirical without any mathematical foundation, it correlates well with survival in multiple injured subjects [19, 20, 22].

Limitations include its reliance on the noninterval AIS, its consideration of injuries with equal AIS scores to be of equal severity regardless of body region, and its exclusion of all but the most serious injury to any body region [21]. Nonetheless, ISS remains the most frequently used summary measure of severity of anatomical injuries.

Anatomic profile

Limitations of the ISS and the growing need for greater precision in quantifying injury so that comparison of groups with similar injuries would be possible, prompted the development of a four-valued Anatomic Profile (AP) [23-25].

Clinical knowledge and research findings regarding the primacy of injuries to the head and chest to mortality [26, 8] motivated the grouping of injuries into components. In the AP, the A-component summarizes all serious (AIS $\geq$ 3 and AIS $<$ 6) head, brain and spinal cord injuries, the B-component considers serious (AIS $\geq$ 3 and AIS $<$ 6) injuries to the front of the neck and the thorax, the C-component covers all other serious injuries, and the D-component is a summary score for all injuries, that are considered nonserious (AIS $<$ 3). Patients with injuries that are

Table 5. Anatomic Profile based on AIS90 [17]

Component	Trauma Description		AIS
	Injury and Region	*AIS 6-Digit Code*	
A	head (without face)	starting with 1	3-4-5
	spinal cord	starting with 63 or 64	3-4-5
B	thorax	starting with 4	3-4-5
	front of neck	starting with 3	3-4-5
C	all other injuries	starting with 2, 5, 7, 8, 9 or starting with 6 and second digit different from 3 or 4	3-4-5
D	all other injuries		1-2

AP component (A, B, C, D) value calculation: $\sqrt{\sum (\text{AIS})^2}$

considered currently not treatable (AIS 6) are not evaluated by AP; they are defined as a "set-aside" group. Whereas ISS only takes into account the most severe injuries in the most severely injured body regions, the AP takes all severe injuries into account.

The AP component values are calculated as the square root of the sum of squares of the AIS scores for all associated injuries. Weighting the values of additional injuries in this way makes the AP more precise than the ISS in describing anatomical injuries. It has been documented that patients with the same ISS but different AP values have markedly different survival probabilities, while the opposite was not true, revealing that the AP describes combined anatomical injuries more precisely than the ISS does [27].

Originally based on AIS85 [28], some modifications of AP have been necessary as a result of the new AIS90 in which the AIS value of some injuries have changed. Table 5 shows the modified AP based on AIS90 [27].

Injury Impairment Scale

At the moment the AIS is accepted as the foundation of nearly all universally applied anatomical injury severity (threat to life) scaling systems. Based on the injury descriptions in AIS90, since 1994 a completely new anatomical injury severity (impairement) scaling system has become available: the Injury Impairment Scale (IIS).

Like the AIS, the IIS is an expertise and consensus-derived, anatomically based system that classifies injuries by body region on an ordinal scale. The scale ranges from IIS 0 to IIS 6. The assessment is meant for previously healthy young adults (25-30 years old) who have received timely and appropriate care and have survived the initial injury without any complications from treatment. Points assigned to each injury should reflect the overall impairment of bodily function at 1 year after single injury in at least 80% of survivors. It is recognized that some injuries may have impairments in a minority of patients (< 20%) that may differ substantially from the IIS scores [29].

Impairment levels have been described as follows:
0 = normal function; no impairment;
1 = impairment detectable but does not limit normal function;
2 = impairment level compatible with most but not all normal functions;
3 = impairment level compatible with some normal functions;
4 = impairment level significantly impedes some normal functions;
5 = impairment level precludes most useful function;
6 = impairment level precludes any useful function.

Although each numerical code has a description attached to it, reliance on the numerical ranking is more important than the description.

Until today, several efforts have been made to validate the IIS against different criterion variables [30-34]. Only two of these studies [32, 34] have tried to validate the IIS in multiple injured patients that have been followed for at least 1 year. They were not able to demonstrate any clinical useful correlation between IIS and impairment.

Applications of trauma severity scores

The main goal of acute trauma care is first to reduce mortality and morbidity and, secondly, to provide the care that will lead to the injured person's maximal functional recovery, that is, to minimize the effects of the injury. The major challenge to health care providers dealing with a trauma patient is to determine rapidly the nature and extent of a patient's injuries and to provide quickly the proper treatment. Severity scaling can be helpful in triage as well as in assessing the quality and effectiveness of trauma care.

Triage

Triage is the classification of patients according to medical needs. As pointed out earlier, only physiological scores are suitable for field-triage purposes, because precise determination of anatomical damage is usually not possible at the scene of injury. Triage can be done to determine the level of trauma care to which the patient needs to be transported, to help in the decision to interhospital transfer, and is done in disaster medicine to identify and prioritize patients who will derive the most medical benefit from treatment.

The RTS is currently the best and most universal physiological trauma scoring system used for triage purposes. However, it should be clear that this scale is not perfect. A recent European study [13] showed that although the possibility of severe injuries increases with the lowering of the RTS, a substantial proportion of the patients who are trauma centre candidates, according to different definitions, have a normal RTS (low sensitivity) (Table 6).

Table 6. Estimates of sensitivity, specificity and predictive values of the RTS

Definition	Sensitivity[a]	Specificity[b]	Predictive value[c] of a negative test	Predictive value[d] of a positive test
ISS[e] ≥18	38%	94%	96%	27%
ISS ≥20	56%	94%	98%	25%
major emergency therapy[f]	76%	94%	99%	25%

[a] Percentage of patients with major injuries (according to the definition used) diagnosed by a lowered RTS
[b] Percentage of patients with only minor injuries (according to the definition used) with a maximum RTS
[c] Percentage of patients with only minor injuries (according to the definition used) among those with a maximum RTS
[d] Percentage of patients with major injuries (according to the definition used) among those with a lowered RTS
[e] ISS calculations based on the Hospital Trauma Index [61]
[f] Emergency thoracotomy, laparotomy, neurosurgery, immediate admission to an intensive care unit or death within 48 h

Quality assessment

To assess the quality of total clinical technical trauma care, the most obvious and probably the most important parameter is the survival of the patient. However, survival is not only the result of the quality of care delivered but is, first of all, a function of the severity of the injuries sustained, the physical condition of the patient before the accident and the time elapsed between the accident and the start of care deliverance. This means that given the same care, the probability of survival of each patient will be different. As a result, unweighted mortality rates are not useful to assess quality of care. However, based on quantified information about the anatomical and physiological condition of each patient, it is possible to calculate the probability of survival of individual patients. Based on these probabilities, one can assess the quality of individual trauma care and performance of trauma care systems.

The two logistic regression models that have been developed for the calculation of the probability of survival in trauma patients are: the "Trauma and Injury Severity Score" (TRISS) [35] model and "A Severity Characterization of Trauma" (ASCOT) [36] model. In both models anatomical as well as physiological scores are incorporated. The anatomical scores account for the anatomical severity of the injuries sustained. In addition to the quantified anatomical severity, the physiological scores account for the physical condition of the patient (i.e., the physiological score of a patient with a bad physical condition will be worse than that of a patient with a good physical condition who has sustained the same injuries). Physiological scores have the potential to change over time, meaning that the first physiological score obtained is also partially determined by the time elapsed between incident and first (para)medical assessment (start of care).

Trauma and Injury Severity Score

Based on the type of injury (blunt or penetrating), patient age, RTS, AIS, and ISS it is possible to calculate a patient's probability of survival. This TRISS methodology [35] is the state-of-the-art trauma outcome evaluation system promoted by the American College of Surgeons Committee on Trauma and applied in the U.S. Major Trauma Outcome Study (MTOS) [37].

TRISS is based on the logistic model:

$$Ps = 1/(1 + e^{-b})$$

where: *Ps* = probability of survival; *e* = 2.7183 (base of Napierian logarithms); *b* = bo + bl (RTS) + b2 (ISS) + b3 (A); *RTS* = Revised Trauma Score at first medical contact; *ISS* = Injury Severity Scale based on a complete description of all anatomical injuries; *A* = age value, patient age $\leq$54 $\Rightarrow$ A = 0, patient age $\geq$55 $\Rightarrow$ A = 1; and where the TRISS values for weighted coefficients[1] [38] depend on the type of injury:
- blunt: (b_0) –0.4843; (b_1) 0.8234; (b_2) –0.0848; (b_3) –1.8084;
- penetrating: (b_0) –1.9127; (b_1) 0.9066; (b_2) –0.0744; (b_3) –0.9637;

– exception: for patients <15 years of age, one always uses coefficients for blunt injury.

TRISS based norms can be used as indicators for institutional quality management. This method is known as the Preliminary Outcome-based Evaluation (PRE) [39]. In PRE the RTS (Y-axis) and ISS (X-axis) are plotted on a graph called the PRE-chart (Fig. 1). Separate PRE-charts are developed for each age and injury-type group.

Although PRE can be used to provide the basis for an internal peer review, a trauma centre, it does not allow comparison of the performance of a hospital against a standard or "norm". The Definitive Outcome-based Evaluation (DEF) [39] was created for this purpose.

In DEF, a Z statistic, which is based on the central limit theorem and the normal approximation to the binomial distribution (without continuity correction), is used to compare the actual number (A) of survivors in a hospital with the expected number, based on current norms.

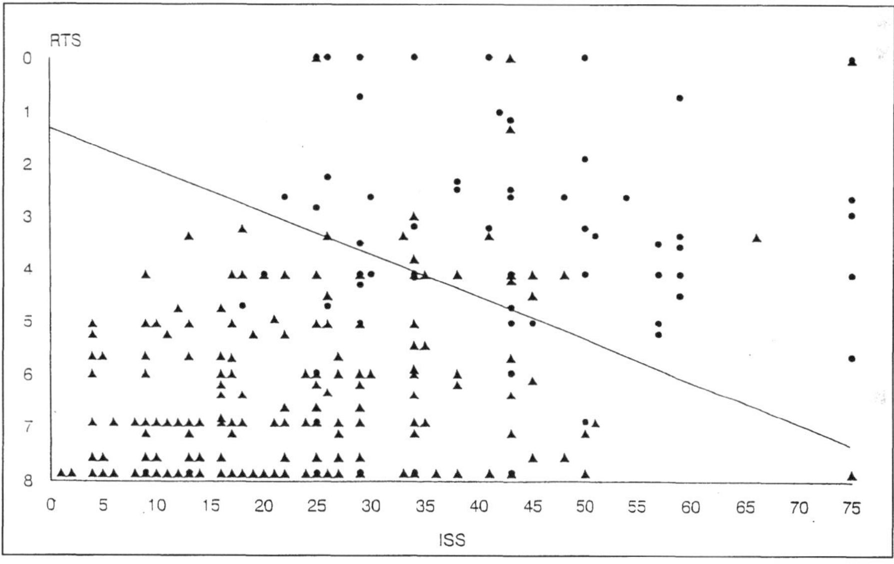

Fig. 1. TRISS PRE-chart. Subgroup: blunt trauma age <55 years. The diagonal line across the chart (PsS0 isobar) marks a Ps of 0.5 for the particular age and injury-type cohort. Patients can be plotted on the PRE-chart as death (*dot*) or alive (*triangle*) and patients with "unexpected outcomes" (survivors above or nonsurvivors below the PsS0 isobar) can be visualized. These cases are believed to need peer review

---

[1] Coefficients are based on Walcer-Duncan logistic regression in a norm data-set of 13 406 patients treated between 1982 and 1989 in four level-1 trauma centres in the US and recoded in 1993 using AIS90.

$$Z = \frac{\left(A - \sum_{i=1}^{n} Ps_i\right)}{\sqrt{\sum_{i=1}^{n} (Ps_i \cdot [1 - Ps_i])}} = \frac{(A - n\pi)}{\sqrt{n\pi \cdot (1 - \pi)}}$$

where: n size of the sample.

For sample sizes of more than 150 patients, Z values between -1.96 and +1.96 (95% confidence interval) indicate no statistically significant difference ($p<0.05$) between actual numbers of survivors and the "norm". A Z value exceeding +1.96 indicates that a statistically significant number of patients survived than which was greater expected by the "norm" and a Z value less than -1.96 indicates the opposite which was greater.

The power of the Z statistic increases with sample size. This means that statistically significant Z values may result from slight but statistically discernible differences between actual and expected number of survivors.

The W statistic provides deeper insight on the clinical significance of statistically significant Z values.

$$W = \frac{\left(A - \sum_{i=1}^{n} Ps_i\right)}{(n/100)} = \frac{(A - n\pi)}{(n/100)}$$

where: A and n are defined as in Z.

W is the number of survivors more (positive W value) or less (negative W value) than would be expected from norm predictions per 100 patients.

Both Z and W are influenced by differences in severity mix between a facility patient data-set and the "norm". Therefore it is also important to know the severity correlation between the data-set and the "norm". The heuristic statistic M expresses this severity correlation on a scale of 0 (poor correlation) to 1 (best correlation) and provides an indicator of the relative bias of the Z statistic. To make an example, this prevents a facility that treats a high proportion of severely injured patients from being falsely labeled as a care provider worse than a facility with less severely injured patients.

M compares the fraction of patients (Fl...F6) falling into each of the six increments of Ps for the "norm" group with the corresponding fraction (Gn...G6) for the study sample. Let Sj be the smallest of the two values Fj and Gj. Then Sl...S6 are summed to arrive at M (Table 7).

$$M = \sum_{i=1}^{6} (S_j)$$

where: S_j minimum (F_j, G_j).

Values of M <0.88 indicate a disparity in the severity match between the groups. Z and W values associated with lower values of M should be viewed with some scepticism.

Table 7. Example of M

Ps range	Number of patients within the Ps range	Fraction of patients within the Ps range		
Age		*Study sample* Gj	*Study sample* Fj	*US norm group* Sj
0.96 - 1.00	2349	0.882	0.828	0.828
0.91 - 0.95	150	0.056	0.045	0.045
0.76 - 0.90	71	0.027	0.044	0.027
0.51 - 0.75	29	0.011	0.029	0.011
0.26 - 0.50	20	0.007	0.017	0.007
0.00 - 0.25	44	0.017	0.036	0.017
Σ	2663	1.000	1.000	**M = 0.935**

Ps, probability of survival

The M statistic is useful for revealing gross differences in injury severity mix, without telling anything about the direction of mismatch. Although the match in injury severity mix is reflected to some extent by the M statistic, this cannot be incorporated into DEF. Therefore, the standardized W (Ws) and Z (Zs) score was introduced [40].

$$W_s = \sum_{i=1}^{6} (W_j \cdot F_j)$$

where: F_j fraction of patients in norm dataset in interval j

$$W = \frac{\left(A_j - \left[\sum_{i=1}^{n_j} Ps_i\right]_j\right)}{(n_j/100)}$$

where: A_j actual number of survivors in interval j and n_j number of actual cases in interval j.

W_s represents the W score that would have been observed if the case mix of injury severities was identical to that of the "norm" dataset.

Z_s, the score measuring the significance of Ws is given by:

$$Z_s = \frac{\sum_{i=1}^{6} (W_j \cdot F_j)}{\sqrt{\sum_{i=1}^{6} VAR\,(W_j) \cdot F_j^2}} \quad \text{where VAR}\,(W_j) = \frac{\left(\sum_{i=n}^{n_j} [Ps_i \cdot (1 - Ps_i)]\right)_j}{(n_j/100)^2}$$

22   L.A. Van Camp, H. Delooz

or:

$$Z_s = \frac{W_s}{SE(W_s)} \qquad \text{where: } SE(W_s) = \sqrt{\sum_{i=1}^{6} VAR\,(W_j) \cdot F_j^2}$$

Table 8 is an illustration of the calculation of Ws and Zs for a sample of 2288 trauma patients, of which 98 died.

A severity characterization of trauma

The limitations of the anatomical component ISS used in TRISS, prompted the development of the AP. As a result ASCOT [36] was developed as a more statistically reliable predictor of Ps than TRISS. ASCOT combines values of the GCS (G), systolic blood pressure (S) and respiratory rate (R), as coded by the RTS (Table 4) with AP components (A, B, and C), patient age, and type of injury.

ASCOT is based on the logistic model:

$$P_s = 1\,/(1 + e^{-k})$$

Table 8. Calculation of Ws and Zs (n=2288)

Ps range	Number of patients	Number of survivors	Expected number of survivors	Contribution to SE(W)	Fraction of patients
	n_j	A_j	$(\Sigma Psi)j$	$(\Sigma[Psi\,(1-Psi)])j$	G_j
0.96-1.00	1974	1960	1948.858	24.594	0.863
0.91-0.95	150	137	141.808	7.718	0.066
0.76-0.90	71	62	60.770	8.633	0.031
0.51-0.75	29	18	19.626	6.232	0.013
0.26-0.50	20	8	7.794	4.642	0.009
0.00-0.25	44	5	3.361	2.900	0.019
	2288	2190	2182.218	54.720	1.000

W for interval = W_j	Fraction of US norm group	Contribution to W_s	Variance of W_j = VAR(W_j)	Contribution to SE(W_s)	Contribution to M
$\dfrac{(A_j - (\Sigma Psi]i)}{(nj/100)}$	F_j	$W_j \cdot F_j$	$\dfrac{(\Sigma Psi\,(1 - Psi)])j}{(nj/100)2}$	$\sqrt{\Sigma\,VAR(Wj)\,Fj}$	S_j
0.564	0.828	0.467	0.063	0.043	0.828
-3.206	0.045	-0.144	3.430	0.007	0.045
1.732	0.044	0.076	17.125	0.033	0.031
-5.607	0.029	-0.163	74.103	0.062	0.013
1.032	0.017	0.018	116.048	0.034	0.009
3.725	0.036	0.134	14.981	0.019	0.019
	1.000		Ws = 0.388	SE(Ws) = $\sqrt{0.199}$	M = 0.945

$Z_s = W_s\,/\,SE(W_s) = 0.388: \sqrt{0.199} = 0.870$

where: P_s = probability of survival; e = 2.7183 (base of Napierian logarithms); k = ko+klG+k2S+k3R+k4A+ksB+k6C+k7Age value; G = value for GCS as coded in RTS at first medical contact; S= value for systolic blood pressure as coded in RTS at first medical contact; R= value for respiratory rate as coded in RTS at first medical contact A, B and C are AP components; and where the ASCOT values for weighted coefficients[2] [27, 38] depend on the type of injury:
– blunt: (k_0) -1.1570; (k_1) 0.7705; (k_2) 0.6583; (k_3) 0.2810; (k_4)-0.3002; (k_5) -0.1961; (k_6) -0.2086; (k_7)-0.6355
– penetrating: (k_0) -1.1350; (k_1) 1.0626; (k_2) 0.3638; (k_3) 0.3332; (k_4) -0.3702; (k_5) -0.2053; (k_6) -0.3188; (k_7) -0.8365.

In ASCOT patient age is modelled more precisely, using, not a binary classification as in TRISS, but a 5-point scale that further breaks down the 54-85 year age group:
- patient age <54 $\Rightarrow$ Age value = 0;
- patient age 55-64 $\Rightarrow$ Age value = 1;
- patient age 65-74 $\Rightarrow$ Age value = 2;
- patient age 75-84 $\Rightarrow$ Age value = 3;
- patient age ≥85 $\Rightarrow$ Age value = 4.

ASCOT's reliance on the AP rather than the ISS to quantify anatomical severity in a more comprehensive way, by incorporating all severe injuries, and its appropriate weighting, not only of the anatomical score, but also of the RTS variables, according to aetiology (blunt or penetrating) of injury, facilitate better severity characterization. The Hosmer-Lemeshow goodness of fit statistics indicates that ASCOT is a more reliable predictor of outcome than TRISS [27].

Patients with very severe (AIS = 6) or very minor (AP components A,B and C = 0) injury are not evaluated by the ASCOT logistic model. These set-aside patient groups are defined, and their respective probabilities of survival are given in Table 9.

Table 9. ASCOT set-asides and their Ps

Maximum AIS	RTS	Type of Injury	Ps
6	0	blunt	0.000
6	0	penetrating	0.000
6	>0	blunt	0.229
6	>0	penetrating	0.222
<6	0	blunt	0.014
<6	0	penetrating	0.026
≤2	>0	blunt	0.998
≤2	> 0	penetratin	0.999

Ps, probability of survival

---

[2] Coefficients are based on Walker-Duncan logistic regression in a norm data-set of 13 406 patients treated between 1982 and 1989 in four level-l trauma centres in the U.S. and recoded in 1993 using AIS90.

The same Z, W, M, Ws and Zs statistics as explained for TRISS can be performed, based on the survival probabilities calculated with ASCOT.

Relevance of TRISS and ASCOT based quality management

For local (institution) audit

TRISS and ASCOT are methods to focus the attention of auditors on a selected number of cases. The following considerations should be made, however, before coming to conclusions.

First, it is important to realize that every "unexpected outcome" is not really unexpected and does not have to mean that the trauma system didn't work properly. For example, if 10 patients all have a Ps of 0.7, one must expect 3 of them to die. "Unexpected outcomes" are a statistical phenomenon and need to be peer-reviewed before conclusions are made.

Secondly, TRISS and ASCOT based quality management that is only based on outcome parameters "death" or "alive" at discharge is very rudimentary. Other outcome parameters are also important, such as length of hospital stay, the frequency of serious complications, medical and other cost of trauma, impairment and disability. However, based on trauma severity scoring, there are no universal methodologies established yet to evaluate these outcome parameters.

For regional, national and European audit

Z, W, M, Ws and Zs statistics, based on TRISS or ASCOT "norms", are very well suited for the assessment of institutional, regional and/or national and international trauma care. However, current TRISS and ASCOT norms are based on data from hospitals in the US.

As norms are dynamic as well as geographically defined (infrastructure, knowledge, and possibilities at a certain time and place), it is possible that the US norms are not suited for the European situation.

First of all, there is an important difference between the European and the USprehospital care. In the US, with the exception of some local initiatives, no medical doctors are involved in delivering prehospital care. The care at the site of the accident and during transport is provided by emergency technicians and paramedics. In many European countries, ambulance crews can call for medical assistance on scene and during transport. As a consequence the quality assessment of the medical care should not be based on the physiological parameters at the moment of hospital admission, but on these parameters measured at the moment of first involvement of the medical team.

Secondly, there is a difference in the population density between the US and Europe. The high density of the European population makes it theoretically possible for ambulances to reach trauma victims sooner than would be possible in the US This might imply that in Europe more trauma patients would survive, but it does not mean that European norms have to be more stringent than the US norms. Since US norms are only based on patients entering the hospital alive, one could be confronted with a higher "hospital trauma mortality"[3] in Europe as a result of a higher number of severe trauma patients reaching the hospital alive and/or getting medical care at the scene.

The structural differences between the US and Europe can also have an influence on the predictive value and significance of the RTS (coded values). In a recent study conducted in the Netherlands, Roorda et al. [13] state that the low sensitivity of the RTS as a triage instrument in the Dutch prehospital setting, in comparison with the U.S., could be the result of the time at which the RTS is measured. As the RTS is dynamic it is possible that in a setting with short prehospital intervention times the RTS, at first survey, does not yet reflect the amount of blood loss, or the severity of secondary brain injuries.

Finally, epidemiologic literature [41-45] states that the causes of trauma and the resulting profile of the injuries in the US are different from those in Europe. This can also have an influence on the validity of the US norm.

Therefore it is important to set-up "Major Trauma Outcome Studies" in Europe in order to establish European and national "norms" which can be used for national and European performance measurement and quality assessment.

Injury epidemiology

One of the core functions in injury control is the collection and analysis of data about injuries in order to document where, when and how injuries occur, what are the risk factors, who is affected and what is the severity. This critical information related to patient's outcome is needed to design, implement and evaluate preventive interventions.

Basic epidemiologic trauma data include information on the distribution of severity, mortality and morbidity associated with each of the causes of injury. Universal anatomic severity scores are essential for severity description in such databases. Only the use of such systems will allow injury epidemiologists to compare trauma patients, to measure preventive interventions and to share the findings of multiple studies.

Conclusions

Changes in trauma care management and the evolution in injury coding mandate the continual updating of relationships between severity measures and outcome. This is crucial because conclusions regarding patient management or health care policy issues should be based, to a large degree, on these data.

---

[3] By "hospital trauma mortality" we mean the mortality of trauma patients after the start of medical care deliverance pre- or in-hospital.

References

1. World Health Organisation and Commonwealth Department of Human Services and Health (1969) Melbourne Declaration On Injury Prevention and Control. Adopted during the Third International Conference on Injury Prevention and Control. WHO, Melbourne
2. U.S. Department of Health and Human Services, Centers for Disease Control, National Center for Environmental Health and Injury Control (1991) Injury Control: position papers from the Third National Injury Control Conference. CDC, Denver
3. Jennett B, Teasdale G, Braakman R et al (1976) Predicting outcome in individual patients after severe head injury. Lancet 1:1031
4. Champion HR, Sacco WJ, Hannan DS (1980) Assessment of injury severity: the Triage Index. Clit Care Med 8:201-208
5. Champion HR, Sacco WJ, Carnazzo AJ et al (1981) Trauma Score. Crit Care Med 9:672-676
6. Champion HR, Gainer PS, Yackee E (1986) A progress report on the Trauma Score in predicting a fatal outcome. J Trauma 26: 927-931
7. Champion HR, Sacco WJ (1984) The Trauma Score as applied to penetrating injury. Ann Emerg Med 13: 415-418
8. Champion HR, Sacco WJ, Copes WS et al (1989) A revision of the Trauma Score. J Trauma 29:623-629
9. Knopp R, Yanegri A, Kallsen G et al (1988) Mechanism of injury in anatomic injury as criteria for prehospital trauma triage. Ann Emerg Med 17:895-902
10. Kreis DJ, Fine EG, Gomez GA et al (1988) A prospective evaluation of field categorization of trauma patients. J Trauma 28:995-1000
11. Morris JA, Auerbach PS, Marshall GA et al (1986) The Trauma Score as a triage tool in the prehospital setting. JAMA 256:1319-1325
12. Emerman CL, Shade B, Kubincanek J (1991) A Comparison of EMT Judgment and Prehospital Trauma Triage Instruments. J Trauma 31:1369-1375
13. Roorda J, van Beek EF, Stapert JWJL, ten Wolde W (1996) Evaluation performance of the Revised Trauma Score as a triage instrument in the prehospital setting. lnjury 27:163-167
14. Harviel JD, Landsman J, Greenberg A et al (1989) The effect of autopsy on injury severity and survival probability calculations. J Trauma 29:766-773
15. Strothert JC Jr, Gbaanador GBM, Herndon DN (1990) The role of autopsy in death resulting from trauma. Journal of Trauma 30:1021-1026
16. American Medical Association Committee on Medical Aspects of Automotive Safety (AMA CMAAS) (1971) Rating the severity of tissue damage. I. The abbreviated scale. JAMA 215:277-280
17. Association for the Advancement of Automotive Medicine (AAAM) (1990) Abbreviated Injury Scale. 1990 revision. AAAM, Des Plaines
18. MacKenzie EJ, Newman AC, Sacco WJ et al (1997) ICDMAP-90 Software User's Guide. The Johns Hopkins University Center for Injury Research and Policy and Tri-analytics, Inc, Bel Air
19. Baker S, O'Neill B, Haddon W et al (1974) The Injury Severity Score: a method for describing patients with multiple injuries and evaluating emergency medicine. J Trauma 14:187-196
20. Baker SP, O'Neill B (1976) The Injury Severity Score: an update. J Trauma 16:822-885

21. Copes WS, Champion HR, Sacco WJ et al (1988) The Injury Severity Score revised. J Trauma 28:69-77
22. Bull JP (1975) The Injury Severity Score of road traffic casualties in relation to mortality, time of death, hospital treatment time and disability. Accident Analysis and Prevention 7:249-255
23. Sacco WJ, Jameson JW, Copes WS et al (1988) Progress toward a new injury severity characterization: injury profiles. Comput Biol Med 18:419-429
24. Copes WS, Sacco WJ, Champion HR et al (1989) Progress in characterizing anatomic injury. 33rd Annual Proceedings, Association for the Advancement of Automotive Medicine, Des Plaines
25. Copes WS, Champion HR Sacco WJ et al (1990) Progress in characterizing anatomic injury. J Trauma 30:1200-1207
26. Gennarelli TA, Champion HR, Sacco WJ et al (1989) Head injury mortality in trauma centers. J Trauma 29:1193-1202
27. Champion HR, Copes WS, Sacco WJ et al (1996) Improved predictions from A Severity Characterization of Trauma (ASCOT) over Trauma and Injury Severity Score (TRISS): Results of an independent evaluation. J Trauma 40:42-49
28. American Association for Automotive Medicine, now Association for the Advancement of Automotive Medicine (AAAM) (1985) Abbreviated Injury Scale. 1985 revision. AAAM, Des Plaines
29. Association for the Advancement of Automotive Medicine (AAAM) (1994) Injury Impairment Scale. AAAM, Des Plaines
30. von Koch M, Nygren A, Tingvall C (1994) Validation of the new Injury Impairment Scale. 38th Annual Proceedings, Association for the Advancement of Automotive Medicine, Des Plaines
31. Yates D.W, Woodford M, Campbell F (1994) Preliminary validation study of the Injury Impairment Scale. 38th Annual Proceedings, Association for the Advancement of Automotive Medicine, Des Plaines
32. Van Camp L, Deschamps M, Sabbe M et al (1996) Assessment of the predictive validity of the Injury Impairment Scale in multiple injured patients with a head injury. 40th Annual Proceedings, Association for the Advancement of Automotive Medicine, Des Plaines
33. Massoud SN, Wallace WA (1996) The Injury Impairment Scale in pelvic and lower limb fractures sustained in road traffic accidents. Injury 27:107-110
34. Waller JA, Skelly JM, Davis JH (1995) The Injury Impairment Scale as a measure of disability. J Trauma 39:949-954
35. Boyd CR, Tolson MA, Copes WS (1987) Evaluating trauma care: the TRISS method. J Trauma 27: 370-378
36. Champion HR, Copes WS, Sacco WJ et al (1990) A new characterization of injury severity. J Trauma 30:539-546
37. Champion HR, Copes W.S, Sacco WJ et al (1990) The Major Trauma Outcome Study: establishing national norms for trauma care. J Trauma 30:1356 -1365
38. Lawnick M (1993) Personnal communication, Washington DC
39. Champion HR, Sacco WJ, Hunt TK (1983) Trauma severity scoring to predict mortality. World J Surgery 7:4-11
40. Hollis S, Yates DW, Woodford M, Foster P (1995) Standardized comparison of performance indicators in trauma: a new approach to case-mix variation. J Trauma 38:763-766
41. Gorman DF, Teanby DN, Sinha MP et al (1995) The epidemiology of major injuries in Mersey Region and North Wales. Injury 26:51-54

42. McNicholl B, Cooke RS (1995) The epidemiology of major trauma in Northern Ireland. Ulster Medical Journal 64:142-146
43. Centers for Disease Control (1995) Emergency department surveillance for weapon-related injuries Massachusetts, November 1993 - April 1994. Morbidity and Mortality Weekly Report 44:160-163
44. Ozonoff VV, Barbec CW, Spivak H et al (1994) Weapon-related injury surveillance in the emergency department. Am J Public Health 84:2024-2025
45. Sauaia A, Moore FA, Moore EE et al (1995) Epidemiology of trauma deaths: a reassessment. J Trauma 38:185-193
46. Williams RE, Schamadan JL (1969) The SIMBOL rating and evaluating system: a measurement tool for injury persons. Arizona Med 16:886-887
47. Kirkpatrick JR, Youmans RL (1971) Trauma Index: an aid in evaluation of injury victims. J Trauma 11:711-714
48. American Medical Association Committee on Medical Aspects of Automotive Safety (AMA CMAAS) (1972) Rating the severity of tissue damage. II. The Comprehensive Injury Scale. JAMA 220:717-720
49. Cowley RA, Sacco WJ, Gill W, et al (1974) A prognostic index for severe trauma. J Trauma 14:1029-1035
50. Champion HR, Sacco WJ, Long W et al (1974) Indicators for early haemodialysis in multiple trauma. Lancet 1:1125-1127
51. Teasdale G, Jennett B (1974) Assessment of coma and impaired consciousness. A practical scale. Lancet 2:81-83
52. Cullen DJ, Civetta JM, Briggs BA et al (1974) Therapeutic Intervention Scoring System: a method for quantitative comparison of patient care. Crit Care Med 2:57-60
53. Keene AR, Cullen DJ (1983) Therapeutic Intervention Scoring System: update 1983. Crit Care Med 11:1-3
54. Bever DL, Veenker CH (1979) An illness severity index for non-physician emergency medical personnel. EMT Journal 3:45-49
55. Sacco WJ, Milholland AV, Ashman WP et al (1977) Trauma indices. Comput Biol Med 7:9-20
56. Goldfarb MA, Ciurey TF, McAslan TC et al (1975) Tracking respiratory therapy in trauma patients. Am J Surg 129:255-258
57. Siegel JH, Cerra FB, Moody EA, et al (1980) The effect on survival of critically ill and injured patients of an ICU teaching service organized about a computer based physiologic CARE system. J Trauma 20:558-579
58. Mayer T, Matlak ME, Johnson DG et al (1980) The modified injury severity scale in pediatric multiple trauma patients. J Pediatr Surg 15:719-726
59. Mayer T, Walker MI, Clark P (1984) Further experience with the modified Abbreviated Injury Severity scale. J Trauma 24:31-34
60. Champion HR, Sacco WJ, Lepper RL (1980) An anatomic index of injury severity. J Trauma 20:197-202
61. American College of Surgeons Commitee on Trauma (ACSCT) (1980) Field categorisation of trauma patients and Hospital Trauma Index, Bull Am Coll Surg 2: 28-33
62. Knaus WA, Zimmerman JE, Wagner DP, et al (1981) APACHE-Acute Physiology and Chronic Health Evaluation: a physiologically based classification system. Critical Care Medicine 9:591 597
63. Moore EE, Dunn EL, Moore JB et al (1981) Penetrating Abdominal Trauma Index. J Trauma 21:399-444
64. Somers RL (1982) New ways to use the 1980Abbreviated Injury Scale - the Probability of Death Score (PODS). Intermal report. Laboratory for Public Health and Health economics, University of Odense

65. Gormican SP (1982) CRAMS scale: field triage of trauma victims. Ann Emerg Med 11:132-135
66. Gregory RT, Gould R.J, Peclet M et al (1985)The mangled extremity syndrome (MES): a severity grading system for multisystem injury of the extremity. J Trauma 25:1147-1150
67. Knaus WA, Draper EA, Wagner DP et al (1985) APACHE II: a severity of disease classification system. Crit Care Med 13:818-829
68. Koehler JJ, Baer LJ, Malafa SA et al (1986) Prehospital Index: a scoring system for field triage of trauma victims. Ann Emerg Med 15:178-182
69. Knaus W, Wagner D, Zimmerman JE et al (1989) APACHE III study design: analytic plan for evaluation of severity and outcome in intensive care unit patients. Crit Care Med 17:S169-S221
70. Tepas JJ, Mollitt DL, Talbert JL et al (1987) The Pediatric Trauma Score as a predictor of injury severity. J Pediatr Surg 22:14-18
71. Hershman MJ, Cheadle WG, Kuftinec D et al (1988) An outcome predictive score for sepsis and death following injury. Injury 19:263-266
72. Chang RWS, Jacobs S, Lee B (1988) Predicting outcome among intensive care unit patients using computerised trend analysis of daily APACHE II scores corrected for organ system failure. Intensive Care Med 14:558-566
73. Moore EE, Schackford SR, Pachter HL et al (1989) Organ Injury Scaling: spleen, liver, kidney. J Trauma 29:1664-1666

Chapter 3

Assessing the severity of trauma and the quality of trauma care

G. Berlot, H. Delooz, A. Gullo

Despite major technological and therapeutic advances, in developed countries trauma remains the leading cause of death in patients younger than 30 years of age [1]. In these subjects, mortality shows a trimodal distribution: roughly 50% of patients die within 1 h after the accident due to injuries incompatible with life; preventive measures (i.e., implementation of speed limits, airbags etc.) appear to be the only way to reduce this burden. Another 30% of subjects die within 3-4 h after the trauma: it is likely that the outcome of many of them could have been different with a better triage or a more rapid transfer to specialized centers (so-called regionalization). The remaining patients die in the Intensive Care Units (ICU) days or weeks after the trauma, mainly due to the consequences of head injuries, infection or multiple organ dysfunction syndrome (MODS). Independent of the clinical course, the final outcome of patients in the two latter groups is likely influenced by two different, interacting categories of factors. The first is represented by direct consequences of the injuries, which can be heavily influenced, in various ways, by the quality of care either in the prehospital or in the hospital phase. Good example of the potential effects of trauma care are the reduction of the incidence and severity of secondary brain injury [2], or the early achievement of proposed resuscitation goals [3]. Conversely, the second category of factors cannot be affected by the quality of care, and includes the victim's age and the presence of coexisting disease [4]. Thus, since outcome relies upon multiple factors acting in different time frames, it appears that: a) any consideration of the probability of survival and/or of the quality of care must be based on careful assessment of the trauma-induced anatomic and physiologic alterations and the preexisting organ functional reserve; b) the quality of treatment must be assessed using a methodologic approach aimed at reducing as much as possible any subjective bias of judgement.

Assessing the severity of injury

The categorization of patients according to the severity of the disease has become a cornerstone of daily ICU practice, with the double aim of: 1) supplying prognostic indications, to compare similar patients treated in different ways and 2) evaluating the quality of care. Currently, the most frequently used severity indexes include the Simplified Acute Physiological Score (SAPS II) [5], the Acute Physiology and Chronic Health Evaluation (APACHE) I and II [6,7] and the

Mortality Prediction Models (MPM) [8]. All these indexes are based on the degree of derangement of selected biological variables which are measured within the first 1 or 2 days of ICU admission, and the probability of in-hospital death is derived from their final scores. Although the utility of these indexes was initially questioned in trauma patients, mainly as they do not take into account the severity of injuries nor the variations occurring after the initial period of admission [9], more recent investigations have demonstrated a good prognostic correlation between the APACHE II and other injury-based prognostic indexes [10]. However, despite the large database on which each prognostic index is based, none of them functions as an outcome predictor on an individual basis [11].

To overcome the particular problems presented by trauma patients, a number of severity indexes based on the entity of injuries have been developed. The most offen used one is the Injury Severity Score (ISS), which is calculated by summing the squared highest points measured in the three most severely injured regions of the body, which is subdivided into six parts [12]. The initial scoring system has been reviewed and simplified and an abbreviated form (AIS) has been proposed [13]. An inherent limitation of these systems is in their inability to distinguish between severity of injury and poor quality of care [14]. As an example, a minor splenic rupture missed at the initial evaluation (ISS 2) resulted in a higher score (ISS 4) when massive hemoperitoneum occurred. Moreover, relevant preexisting biological variables, including age and functional status, are not even taken into account.

Other indexes have been developed to describe the pathophysiologic derangements observed during the prehospital phase of trauma care, mainly with the aim of facilitating the on-the-spot triage and assessing the quality of immediate trauma care.

The most widely used are the Trauma Score (TS) and its simplified version, the revised Trauma Score (rTS) [15]. Both systems are based on the sum of points assigned to cardiovascular, respiratory and neurologic variables (measured with the Glasgow Coma Scale) recorded at the scene of the accident.

Assessing the probability of survival in trauma patients

Although this approach has been strongly criticized on the basis of many statistical and methodological shortcomings, in general terms the quality of care is evaluated by measuring the difference between the observed and expected number of deaths, as predicted by one of the many scoring systems available, occurring in a population of patients admitted to a certain ICU with a particular diagnosis [11]. Thus, theoretically, it is possible to identify one or more diagnostic or therapeutic errors which ultimately influence outcome. In trauma care, this task is particularly difficult, as many professionals are involved, each with different levels of skill and/or complexity of task and acting in different time frames.

In the attempt to infer a prognostic indication from the patient's age using the acute trauma-induced physiologic derangements, as expressed by the rTS, and the severity of anatomic injuries, as assessed by the ISS, Boyd et al. [16] developed the

Table 1. The Trauma Score and Injury Severity (TRISS) method

- $PS = 1/(1+e^{-b})$
- Set of coefficients is a b_0, b_1, b_2, b_3 for penetrating and blunt trauma
- Age: score 1 if patient's age is <55, otherwise score 0
- rTS=(GCS coded value · 0.9368) + (systolic blood pressure coded value · 0.7326) +
     (respiratory rate coded value · 0.2908)

PS, probability of survival; e, 2.718 base of natural logarithm; $b = b_0 + b_1$ (rTS) + b_2 (ISS) + b_3 (age)

Trauma Score and Injury Severity Score (TRISS). Its value, which requires a rather complex calculation (Table 1), indicates a probability of survival (PS).

However, this method has been criticized on the basis of several considerations. First, the TRISS-derived PS can be biased by the above mentioned inability of the ISS to distinguish between poor care and severity of injuries. Second, in elderly people the rTS poorly reflects the degree of cardiovascular impairment [17]. Third, when TRISS-evaluated unexpected deaths were reviewed by local committees of experts, it turned that most of them were not unexpected from a clinical point of view [18]. Actually, the falsely good expected outcome was rather due to a sensitivity of 60% for blunt trauma, the underestimation of head injuries, the inability of the ISS to adequately describe the effects of multiple injuries to one body region, and the failure to take into full account the effect of age [18]. To overcome the limitations of the TRISS method, A Severity Characterization of Trauma (ASCOT) has been recently developed [19]. Like TRISS, the ASCOT system uses the measurement of injury severity, age and type of injury, calculated via the rTS and the anatomic profile of injuries, derived from the AIS, to characterize a patient and provide a PS (Table 2). To exclude patients with only minor injuries and to reduce the related background noise, only injuries with an AIS >2 are taken into account.

In comparisons between TRISS and ASCOT, this latter system was demonstrated to be superior [18], but another study failed to confirm these findings, especially when pediatric patients or patients with penetrating injuries were involved [20]. Moreover, the limited advantage provided by the ASCOT is offset by its complexity and the increased necessity of computer-processing. Overall, as far as the misclassification of patients is concerned, the ASCOT was found to be more accurate regarding patients dying after blunt injuries, whereas the TRISS method was associated with significantly less misclassifications regarding survivors of either penetrating or blunt injuries [21]. Another relevant limitation of both TRISS and ASCOT consists in their having been designed for the prediction of mortality as

Table 2. The A Severity Characterization of Trauma (ASCOT) method

---

- $PS = 1/(1+(e)-m)$

    $m = m_0 + m_1G + m_2S + m_3R + m_4a + m_5b + m_6c$

$m_0\text{-}m_6$, values derived from logistic regression analysis of the MTOS database; G, coded GCS value; S, coded systolic pressure value; R, coded respiratory value; $a\text{-}c$, coded anatomic profile (IIS) value the only outcome measure of trauma patients, without supplying any information about resource utilization. This latter issue appears particularly important since the best allocation of resource is becoming a key factor in the management of ICUs. Recently, Rutledge et al. [22] demonstrated that a much simpler scoring system based on the widely used International Classification of Disease (ICISS), was superior to both ISS and TRISS as predictor of in-hospital death, length of stay and overall cost of care. Moreover, this methodology does not involve the time-consuming data processing required by the TRISS. Despite their disadvantages, the TRISS and ASCOT methods are largely used to assess the quality of care, and in many studies a death occurring in patients with a TRISS-calculated PS ≥50% is considered avoidable, needing a more-in-depth investigation to establish its possible cause(s) (missed diagnoses, delayed triage or treatment etc.). However, this approach has been questioned, as it considers potentially rescueable patients with relatively minor injuries who ultimately die due to their chronic medical problems [23]. To overcome this problem, it has been proposed that clinical peer review of the medical documentation of patients who died after trauma could be more accurate in identifying preventable deaths, and possibly in finding out the possible cause(s). However, even this approach is not problem-free: in a recent study, Wilson et al. [24] demonstrated that when review panels of experts were gathered to identify preventable deaths, using three different methods of review and discussing the medical charts, the consensus varied from 10% to 45%, indicating an elevated risk of subjectivity.

At the present time, no prognostic index has been developed that is yet able to predict the outcome of trauma patients with a sensibility and specificity of 100%. Thus, it appears that to evaluate the quality of care it is advisable: a) to identify patients who die despite a low expected risk of death, calculated via the available methods; and b) once this preliminary screening has been performed, to look for undiscovered cause(s) of death. In the absence of such potential causes, the patient should be considered at higher-than-predicted risk for reasons which could not be anticipated by the used index [25].

Epidemiology of the avoidable death in trauma patients

Despite the relevance of the issue, relatively few investigations have addressed the occurrence of errors and preventable deaths among trauma patients, and many of them are difficult to compare due to different definitions of clinical errors, endpoints of the studies and characteristics of the patients enrolled [24]. However, independent of these limitations, it appears that preventable deaths can occur in every postraumatic phase, from the on-site rescue to advanced ICU care. Unfortunately, the published data are controversial, and thus it is difficult to draw established conclusions about the time frame when errors, and consequently preventable deaths, are more likely to occur. As an example, whereas from one study it appeared that the time spent in the prehospital phase to establish an i.v. line and fluid resuscitate the injured patient was associated with an increased rate of preventable death [26], other investigators demonstrated increased survival of patients who needed a prolonged time on the trauma scene due to therapeutic maneuvers, including the insertion of multiple venous lines and the drainage of pneumothoraces [27]. Indeed, these different results appear to emphasize the ongoing controversy existing between the "scoop and run" versus the "stay and play" strategy for the immediate treatment of trauma patients [28]. The same lack of agreement applies to the in-hospital phase. In an Italian study, Stocchetti et al. [29] demonstrated 10% clearly preventable deaths, and another 23% were considered potentially preventable. The cause of the preventable deaths was failure to adequately treat shock and/or hypoxia. In a larger study involving 12,910 patients followed throughout their clinical course, Davis et al. [30] demonstrated that significant errors occurred in 15% of nonsurvivors, and that 50% of deaths could be considered potentially or positively preventable. However, in this study, most errors occurred in the advanced phase, when the patients had been already resuscitated and admitted to the ICU, and were associated mostly with failed recognition and treatment of sepsis and with a lack of prophylaxis of pulmonary thromboembolism in high-risk patients.

Conclusions

As trauma care is compounded by the interaction of multiple specialties, the aim of its quality assessement is to identify and strengthen the weakest link in the chain of care and to reduce, and possibly eliminate, management errors leading to a further worsening of the patients' conditions or even to their deaths. Unfortunately, despite a number of methods developed, this process is far from having reached conclusive results from a methodological point of view, and a gold standard of evaluation is not available yet. As far as the rate of preventable deaths is considered a marker of the quality of care, the predictions supplied by the currently used methods are not sufficiently accurate to be suitable on an individual basis, mainly because not all the physiologic variables influencing outcome are taken into account.

References

1. Trunkey DD (1991) Initial treatment of patients with severe trauma. New Engl J Med 324:1259-1263
2. Chestnut RM, Marshall Lf, Klauber MR et al (1993) The role of secondary brain injury in determining outcome from severe head injury. J Trauma 34:216-222
3. Porter JM, Ivatury RR (1998) In search of the optimal end points of resuscitation in trauma patients: a review. J Trauma 44:908-914
4. Sacco WJ, Copes WS, Bain LW et al (1993) Effect of preinjury illness on trauma patient survival outcome. J Trauma 35:538-543
5. LeGall JR, Lemeshow S, Saulnier F (1993) A new simplified acute physiology score (SAPS II) based on an European/North American multicenter study. JAMA 270:2957-2963

6. Knaus WA, Draper EA, Wagner DP, Zimmermenn JE (1985) APACHE II: a severity of disease classification system. Crit Care Med 13:818-829

7. Knaus WA, Draper EA, Wagner DP et al (1991) The APACHE III prognostic system. Risk prediction of hospital mortality for critically ill hospitalized adults. Chest 100:1619-1636

8. Lemeshow S, Teres D, Klar J, Avrunin JS, Gelblach SH, Rapoport J (1993) Mortality Prediction Models (MPM II) based on an international cohort of intensive care unit patients. JAMA 270:2478-2486

9. Vassar MJ, Wilkerson CL, Duran PJ et al (1992) Comparison of APACHE II, TRISS and a proposed 24 hour ICU point system for prediction of outcome in ICU trauma patients. J Trauma 32:490-499

10. Wong DT, Barrow PM, Gomez M, mcGuire GP (1996) A comparison of the Acute Physiology and Chronic Health Evaluation (APACHE) II score and the Trauma Injury Severity Score (TRISS) for outcome assessment on intensive care unit trauma patients. Crit Care Med 24:1642-1648

11. Moreno R (1998) Performances of the ICU: are we able to measure it? In: Vincent JL (ed) Yearbook of intensive care and emergency medicine. Springer-Verlag, Berlin Heidelberg New York, pp 729-743

12. Baker SP, O'Neil B (1976) The Injury Severity Score: an update. J Trauma 16:882-885

13. Champion HR, Sacco WJ, Copes WS et al (1989) A revision of the trauma score. J Trauma 29:623-629.

14. Rutledge R (1996) The Injury Severity Score is unable to differentiate between poor care and severe injury. J Trauma 40:944-950

15. Klasen HJ, ten Duis HJ, Kingma J (1995) Methods of registration and injury severity score scoring. In: Goris RJA, Trenz O (eds) The integrated approach to trauma care the first 24 hours. Springer-Verlag, Berlin Heidelberg New York pp 13-24

16. Boyd CR, Tolson MA, Copes WS (1987) Evaluating trauma care: the TRISS method. J Trauma 27:370-378

17. Bull JP, Dickson GR (1991) Injury scoring by TRISS and ISS/age. Injury 21:127-131

18. Oestern HJ, Kabus K (1994) Comparison of various trauma score systems. Unfallchirurg 97:177-184

19. Champion HR, Copes WS, Sacco WJ et al (1996) Improved prediction from A Severity Characterization of Trauma (ASCOT) over Trauma and Injury Severity Score (TRISS): result of an independent study. J Trauma 40:42-49

20. Markle J, Cayten CG, Byrne DW, Moy F, Murphy JG (1992) Comparison between TRISS and ASCOT methods in controlling for injury severity. J Trauma 33:326-332

21. Markle J, Cayten CG, Bryne DW et al (1992) Comparison between TRISS and ASCOT methods in controlling for injury severity. J Trauma 31:A1719

22. Rutledge R, Osler T, Emery S, Kromhout Shiro (1998) The end of the Injury Severity Score (ISS) and the Trauma-Injury Severity Score (TRISS): ICISS, an international classification of disease, 9th revision-based prediction tool, outperforms both ISS and TRISS as predictors of trauma patient survival, hospital charges and hospital lenght of stay. J Trauma 44:41-49

23. Pories SE, Gamelli RL, Pilcher DB et al (1989) Practical evluation of trauma deaths. J Trauma 29:1607-1610

24. Wilson DS, McElligot J, Fielding LP (1992) Identification of preventable trauma deaths: counfounded inquiries? J Trauma 32:45-51

25. Karmy-Jones R, Copes WS, Champion HR et al (1992) Results of a multi-institutional outcome assessemnt: results of a structured peer review of TRISS-designated unexpected outcomes. J Trauma 32:196-203

26. Sampalis JS, Boukas S, Lavoie A et al (1995) Preventable death evaluation of the appropriateness of the on-site trauma care provided by Urgences-Santé physicians. J Trauma 39:1029-1035
27. Nardi G, Massarutti D, Muzzi A et al (1994) Impact of emergency medical helicopter service on mortality for trauma in north east Italy: a regional prospective audit. Eur J Emerg Med 1:69-77
28. Bickell WH, Wall MJ, Pepe PE et al (1994) Immediate versus delayed fluid resuscitation for hypotensive patients with penetrating torso injuries. New Engl J Med 331:1105-1109
29. Stocchetti N, Pagliarini G, Gennari M et al (1994) Trauma care in Italy: evidence of in-hospital preventable deaths. J Trauma 36:401-405
30. Davis JW, Hoyt DB, McArdle MS et al (1991) The significance of critical care errors in causing preventable deaths in trauma patients in a trauma system. J Trauma 31:813-819

Chapter 4

Trauma transport

M. LIPP, W.F. DICK

The qualified transport of trauma patients is a challenge for every emergency medical system (EMS). Any transport of a critically ill trauma patient may be associated with acute physiological changes, leading to complications in the cardiovascular system (i.e., insufficient volume substitution causing hypotension, tachycardia, and arrhythmias), the respiratory system (i.e., difficulties in artificial ventilation, resulting in hypercarbia and/or hypoxia), the central nervous system (i.e., increase in intracranial pressure with the consequence of brain edema), the thermoregulation and protection, the metabolic regulation, and the gastrointestinal system [4, 7, 10, 19, 28].

Therefore, well-recognized prerequisites for positive outcome are a well-defined structure, a profound (repeated) training of all team members, and proper medical and technical equipment [6, 11, 12, 16, 27].

Transport tasks may be distinguished between a move:
- from the scene of the accident to a hospital (primary transport);
- within a hospital or between hospitals (secondary transport).

The term "primary transport" describes an immediate transport of medical personnel (emergency physicians and paramedics) to the emergency site within life-saving minutes for treatment and stabilization of casualties at the scene followed by medically supervised transport to an appropriate hospital. Primary transports have absolute priority over any other requests to the EMS [15, 18, 24]. A secondary transport is carried out if a patient has been stabilized and treated in a hospital and then has to be transferred to a specialized center [9, 10, 14, 22, 26]. Both primary and secondary transports are carried out by ground and air rescue systems and have their own specific tasks and resulting structures. In most countries, the personnel and technical infrastructure provided for primary transports is used for secondary transports as well.

For a profound understanding of the trauma transport issue it seems useful to describe system patterns of primary transport first, followed by special structures of secondary transport. This article will focus on a physician-based prehospital system with trained paramedics as assistants: as an example the German system is taken, which is comparable to that of many states. In countries with a paramedic-based EMS, the performance should be compared to the described system.

In not a few European countries, a minimum response interval has to be observed, i.e., an interval which starts at the moment the EMS is alerted and ends at the moment at which the patient receives appropriate care [15]. The response interval ranges from a minimum of 7 min up to a maximum of 15 min.

Structures for primary transport

Medical rescue organizations and fire brigade

As a result of World War II there are different organizations involved in the German EMS: in the formerly American and French controlled areas (southern part of Germany) the German Red Cross is the leading EMS organization, in the British area (north part) the fire brigades are the predominant EMS provider. Overall, up to 37% of all EMS rescue activities are performed by fire brigades, in particular in the cities and in the northern states (more than 60%). The other German medical rescue organizations are different in origin and age. The German Red Cross (DRK) is 130 years old and is part of the International Red Cross Societies. The "Arbeiter-Samariter-Bund" (ASB) was founded in 1889 and has its roots in the workers' movement. Today it is a nonpolitical medical rescue organization, providing EMS in all states of Germany. The "Johanniter Unfall-Hilfe" (JUH) and the "Malteser-Hilfsdienst" (MHD) have their origin in the Protestant and Catholic churches, respectively, and started their activities in the EMS in 1952 and 1953, respectively. Fire brigade and medical rescue organizations provide vehicles and medical equipment, they are also employees of the paramedics, but not of the emergency physicians.

Rescue coordination center

Germany is divided into multiple EMS districts, which are often identical with the political topographic structure of the particular region. Every rescue coordination center (RCC) activates and coordinates within its area all activities of ground rescue vehicles and rescue helicopters. The RCC also coordinates bed availability and the transport of critically ill patients to the appropriate hospitals. The RCC relays information from the rescue team to the receiving hospital or other specialty facilities (i.e., a detoxification center) as necessary. All RCCs are state-controlled institutions, operated by the fire brigade or medical rescue organizations. In the north and most of the new states RCCs coordinate fire brigade and EMS; in the south the services run separate dispatch centers. Most dispatchers are paramedics or fire fighters, a special training for EMS-RCC dispatchers still does not exist.

Communication

Center of the communication process is the RCC. Permanent open telephone lines are established to all rescue stations, the dispatch centers of police and fire departments (only if the EMS runs a separate RCC), as well as major receiving hospitals. Two-way radio communication devices, beepers, and, in some centers, computerized information retrieval systems are used. Emergency calls from various sources, including individuals, police, and fire brigade are channeled to the RCC. The countrywide emergency telephone number is 112 (fire brigade and EMS), but in some parts of Germany the RCC can (also) be reached by dialing different and individual numbers, implemented by medical rescue organizations. This has caused some confusion, and under certain circumstances up to 72% of all emergency calls are not directed primarily to the RCC [17].

Ground vehicles

The various types of EMS ground vehicles include: smaller ambulances, used for transport of noncritically ill patients (KTW); emergency ambulances, primarily designed for the stabilization of critically ill patients (RTW); MICUs, generally dispatched with an emergency physician; and finally, cars designed exclusively for the transport of the emergency physician to the scene (NEF). The medical rescue equipment of the ground rescue vehicles is tailored to the specific roles and specified by law.

Smaller ambulances (KTW), normally used for the transport of noncritically ill patients only, are equipped with a litter, transport chair, oxygen tank, suction device, ventilation masks and bags for artificial respiration, IV infusion supplies, dressings, and bandages. In reality, most of the KTWs are equipped above the minimum requirements. The actual financial situation caused some medical rescue organizations to reduce the equipment again to the legal level. However, BLS resuscitation equipment is found in all ambulances; that makes it possible for the RCCs to dispatch even a KTW as the next available vehicle first, followed by an emergency ambulance (RTW), in an effort to reduce the response time. Most KTWs are dispatched with two semi-trained paramedics (RS).

Emergency ambulances (RTW) are used for on-site emergency care and transport of critically ill patients. They have to be supplied, in addition to the equipment of a KTW, with a vacuum mattress, ECG, and defibrillator, and complete resuscitation kits for adults and children, including endotracheal intubation instruments, surgical instruments and emergency drugs. The crew consists of two fully trained paramedics (RA). Actually, the number of RTWs equipped with semi-automatic defibrillators is increasing: the fire brigade of Hamburg has just implemented these defibrillators on all 63 RTWs.

By law, the equipment of a MICU, which is generally dispatched with a certified emergency physician and two fully trained paramedics (RA), does not differ from the material of RTWs. But, in reality, even the equipment of RTWs exceeds the legal requirements by far: automatic respirators, blood pressure monitors, 12-lead-ECG, pulsoximeters, and capnographs [15, 21].

Cars designed for the transport of the emergency physician to the emergency site (NEF), operating in a so-called "rendezvous system" are equipped with ACLS kits (for adults and children), oxygen, defibrillator/ECG and emergency drugs; they are operated by semi trained paramedics (RA).

Helicopter rescue system

To complement the ground EMS system, there is a network of 48 EMS helicopter stations throughout all parts of Germany (RTH). The helicopter rescue system covers more than 90% of Germany. This system allows a quick response time even in the rural areas, smooth transport of the patient, and rapid transfer to a medical center if necessary [3, 5, 8, 13, 25]. The use of most helicopters is limited by weather and daylight conditions, due to the fact that only a few helicopters of the army and the disaster control are equipped for night flights. The crew consists of a certified emergency physician, a fully trained paramedic (RA), a flight officer and a pilot. The system is not only used for transport of patients after medical treatment at the scene, up to the half of the patients are transported by a ground rescue vehicle after receiving medical treatment by the emergency physician of the helicopter.

The simultaneous dispatching of ground rescue vehicles and a helicopter has been demonstrated to have some advantages. At the emergency site, the paramedics can start to restore or maintain vital functions (i.e., BLS or ACLS). If they arrive earlier, an emergency ambulance provides a dry, warm, well-lit "emergency room" for the initial medical treatment of the patients, a great advantage especially during rough weather conditions.

The helicopters used in the German EMS are generally equipped in the same way as the emergency ambulances as regards the medical aspects. The smallest helicopter operated, BO 105, has a restricted cabin area, and thus stabilization must occur before flight. Newer models (i.e., BK 117 or EC 135) provide an unobstructed cabin area, so that treatment is possible during flight. The Bell UH1D is operated on a "Search and Rescue" principle.

Most of the helicopters have high maneuverability and small external dimensions, and are twin-engine operated. Only a few helicopters, mainly army equipment, are allowed to fly at night. The take-off time after alerting should be less than 2 min. Statistics in 1985 for the helicopter located at Munich showed that the in-flight time after take-off was approximately 10 min, with an average distance of 30 km to the emergency site.

The helicopters are located mainly at major hospitals and operated by the disaster control, the German army, the German automobile association, and a private rescue organization (German Air Rescue). The air rescue system is used as a primary transport facility as well as for secondary transports.

Education and training of EMS personnel

Emergency physicians

In Germany, emergency physicians routinely staff ambulances to render medical treatment to the emergency patient [1, 2, 16]. At the scene, it is the responsibility of the emergency physician to provide the whole range of the necessary medical care to the patient. This consists of all procedures of ATLS and ACLS as well as pain management and invasive procedures. The emergency physician must have knowledge of pathophysiology, symptoms, and treatment of typical emergencies in the specialties of surgery, internal medicine, pediatrics, and anaesthesiology. On the administrative side, emergency physicians must know the structure of the local health and rescue system, i.e., locations, departments, and capabilities of the hospitals in their particular area [2, 11, 12, 18, 20, 27].

In contrast to other countries, Germany has no specific emergency departments within hospitals. Emergency medicine is a component in the education of anesthetists, as well as internal specialists and surgeons. Although anesthetists often meet the demands for emergency physicians best, in Germany, surgeons, internal specialists, pediatricians, and general practitioners also work as emergency physicians.

To ensure standards, physicians have to complete successfully a specialty training program and gain clinical experience of at least 18 months after becoming a specialist, of which 6 months is experience in an intensive care unit. During this period, the techniques of emergency medicine, artificial ventilation, endotracheal intubation, and peripheral and central venipuncture, to name a few, are perfected.

Additionally, an 80 h program on special topics of emergency medicine theory must be successfully completed. Finally, before being certified as an "emergency physician" by the local health authority, the physician must treat at least ten emergency patients in the prehospital setting under the supervision of a senior emergency physician [1, 16, 18].

Paramedics

Before September 1989, a semi-trained paramedic (RS) was trained for 520 h, divided as follows: 160 h of theory, 160 h of practical training in a hospital, 160 h of practical training in an ambulance, and 40 h of a final theory course. After passing a state certification test consisting of oral, written and practical examinations, the candidate is allowed to work. The aim of the described training was to enable the paramedics (RS) to restore or maintain vital functions (i.e., cardiopulmonary resuscitation), but without independent application of drugs and to assist emergency physicians in their treatment. Paramedics (RS), however, had no profession comparable to that of any other workers in the German health system [18].

In September 1989, the education of paramedics was changed fundamentally: the theoretical and practical training at school was extended to a 1 200 h course and an additional 1 600 h of practical education at special ambulance dispatching stations. The training now lasts 2 years and ends with an extensive state certification procedure. Fully trained paramedics (RA) who have achieved this certification are awarded the official professional title "Rettungsassistent."

Paramedics may work as full-time employees (fire brigade and private ambulance companies or medical rescue organizations) or as volunteers (medical rescue organizations only).

Structures for secondary transport

All outlined structures for primary transport may be used for secondary transports, but due to the increasing number of such transports, a seperate system has to be organized [9, 10, 14, 22]:
- ground vehicles with space for intensive monitoring and even treatment during the transport;
- aircraft (helicopters and fixed-wing crafts) for long-range transports;
- coordination centers for secondary transports;
- specially trained physicians and paramedics.

For the training of flight physicians performing secondary intensive care during transport, the DIVI has established a curriculum, containing some specific aspects [6]:

- history and purpose of air medical transport (AMT);
- medical equipment for AMT;
- flight team members/roles;
- guidelines for AMT;
- flight physiology;
- legal and ethical issues;
- transport vehicles;
- practical orientation;
- aircraft and flight safety;
- documentation/TQM.

Although 75% of all secondary transports are performed with ground vehicles, the frequency of air transportation is increasing. In the last few years a net of intensive care transport helicopters has been established in Germany. The decision as to which type of transport vehicle is to be preferred follows the same rules as for primary transport of trauma patients, as outlined below. A major advantage of air transportation is the speed and the possibility to transport patients even during the night with specially equipped helicopters (i.e., MD 900, Bell 222, Bell 412 or SA 365) [8, 12, 25].

Response procedures in the EMS

After taking down the essential and necessary information of an emergency call, the paramedic on duty has to decide which rescue team or vehicle is to be sent out. The activation time of an ambulance after alerting should be less than 45 s.

Emergency calls that describe critically ill patients lead to the notification of an emergency physician, and the specific indications are prioritized at all rescue coordination centers. The transport of the physicians is either carried out by a MICU, normally located at the hospital (compact system), or by a specially designed car (rendezvous system) with the emergency ambulance arriving separately. The compact system is still operated in some cities and towns, whereas the rendezvous system is operated in the most rural areas. In an emergency, three dispatch strategies are used: the "next available vehicle" strategy, the "assignment" strategy, and the "multiple-purposes vehicle" strategy. The "next standing vehicle" strategy means that the rescue vehicle (KTW, RTW or MICU) which is actually nearest to the emergency site has to be alerted, regardless of its configuration or equipment. The main advantage of this principle is the short response time (less than 8.8 min in 85% of all emergencies in the town of Karlsruhe, for example). A disadvantage, however, is that in some cases, critically ill patients have to be treated or even transported in underequipped, small ambulances. The "assignment" strategy means that only emergency ambulances (RTW or MICU) are sent to an emergency patient and the smaller ambulances (KTW) are reserved for nonurgent transport of noncritically ill patients. The advantage of this principle is that patients can be treated with appropriate medical equipment before and during the transport. Disadvantages are the slightly extended response time compared to the "next available vehicle" strategy and the increased costs for the whole emergency medical service [18].

Treatment and tactical considerations

Two principle concepts exist according to which trauma patients are transported from the scene of an accident to the hospital [15]:
– the scoop and run concept;
– the stay, treat and transport concept.

In Europe the latter is most often applied, although occasionally in cases of severe bleeding due to lacerations of the great vessels, the first approach has to be selected. Requirements for a safe tranport need to follow the principles of the "prehospital stay and treat concept", which is an essential part of the total trauma intensive care concept. Thus, careful assessment and resuscitation have to be performed before transport under continuous monitoring and life support by qualified and experienced personnel is initiated.

The decision for a certain medical procedure depends on the type, location, and severity of the given trauma. Typical facts to be considered are:
– hemorrhagic shock;
– acute lung injury;
– lacerations of the great vessels;
– brain trauma;
– chest wall instability;
– severe bone injuries;
– injuries of the vertebral column.

According to type and extent of the injury, the following strategies have to be facilitated:
– airway management with endotracheal intubation as gold standard;
– artificial ventilation;
– establishment of adequate venous access;
– (rapid) volume replacement;
– sedation and/or analgesia;
– anesthesia;
– stabilization of fractures;
– chest tube insertion.

Basic and advanced monitoring, using portable monitors, for trauma patients include (in the prehospital setting and during transport):
– ECG;
– blood pressure (invasive and noninvasive);
– SaO_2;
– endtidal CO_2;
– temperature.

The decision as to which vehicle is preferrable for the given trauma patient depends on various factors, i.e., distance between locations, traffic congestion, urgency of transport, patient comfort, expected complications, and space needed during transport [3-5, 7, 19].

Air transportation is often preferred in trauma patients, but there are some aspects to be considered [5, 7, 14, 19, 22, 23, 26-28].

- Air transport may lead to hypoxia (Table 1) and dysbarism (extension of gas in the abdomen, gut, eye, skull, and chest). The relative gas volume increases with altitude, a given volume (sea level) increases at 1 500 m 1.25 times, at 3 000 m 1.5 times.
- Noise and vibrations may cause distress and anxiety in the conscious patient.
- Strong 3-dimensional forces may affect the patient, especially during bad weather flights.
- Monitoring and treatment may be limited in the cabin (BO 105).

Table 1. Oxygen supplementation required to maintain a PaO_2 of 100 mmHG achieved at sea level by several inspired oxygen concentrations (FiO_2)[a] up to altitudes of 3 000 m

Sea level (%)	Flight level 400 m (%)	Flight level 1 200 m (%)	Flight level 1 800 m (%)	Flight level 2 400 m (%)	Flight level 3 000 m (%)
21	23	25	27	29	32
30	33	35	38	42	45
40	44	47	51	55	60
50	54	59	64	69	75
60	65	70	76	83	90
70	76	82	90	97	100
80	87	94	100		
90	98	100			
100	100				

[a] FiO_2 >60% may require endotracheal intubation

References

1. Ahnefeld FW, Weißauer W, Lippert H-D, Knuth P (1995) Rettungsdienst im Spannungsfeld zwischen Politik, Recht und Medizin. Dtsch Ärztebl 92:A674-A678
2. Ahnefeld FW, Dick W, Schuster HP (1995) Die ärztliche Aufgabenstellung im deutschen Rettungsdienst. Notfallmedizin 21:165-169
3. Anderson TEA, Rose WD, Leicht MJ (1987) Physician staffed helicopter scene response from a rural trauma center. Ann Emerg Med 16:58-61
4. Baxt WG (1985) Prehospital treatment and transport of the trauma patient. In: Baxt WG (ed) Trauma: the first hour. Appleton Century Crofts, East Norwalk, pp 293-303
5. Bollinger CT, Kiener A, Weber W, Reigner M, Ritz R (1990) Helikoptertransport: Streßbelastung für Patienten? Notfallmedizin 16:36-41
6. DIVI (1997) Empfehlungen zur ärztlichen Qualifikation bei Intensivtransporten. Düsseldorf
7. Edlin S (1989) Physiological changes during transport of the critically ill. Intensive Care World 6:131-133
8. Felleiter P (1996) Qualitätsmanagement in der Luftrettung. Notarzt 12:152-157
9. Grande CM, Williams DA, McCauley M (1991) Critical care transport: mobile management of the trauma patient inside and outside the trauma center. In: Stene JK, Grande CM (eds) Trauma anesthesia. William and Wilkins, Baltimore, pp 1011-1042

10. Guidelines Committee of the ACCCM, SCCM, AACCN (1993) Guidelines for the transfer of critically ill patients. Crit Care Med 21:931-937
11. Klingshirn H (1996) Der ärztliche Leiter Rettungsdienst. Notfallmedizin 22:101-103
12. Krohmer JR, Hunt RC, Benson Nbieniek RB (1993) Flight physician training program-core content. Prehosp Disast Med 8:183-184
13. Lampl L, Helm J, Weidringer JW, Winter M (1996) Stellenwert der differenten Formen der Luftrettung im Konzept des Rettungsdienstes. Notarzt 12:145-149
14. Link J, Krause H, Wagner W, Papadopoulos G (1990) Intrahospital transport of critically ill patients. Crit Care Med 18:1427
15. Lipp M (1993) Preclinical emergency medicine systems: international comparisons. Anaesthesist 42:623-629
16. Lipp MDW (1995) Fachkundenachweis "Rettungsdienst". Notfallmedizin 21:37-41
17. Lipp M, Mihaljevic V, Dick W (1994) Analysis of telephone calls placed to Fire Brigade, Emergency Medical Services, and General Practitioners' Emergency Services in an emergency medical service system. Anaesthesist 43:187-193
18. Lipp M, Dick W, Ahnefeld FW, Bartels F, Knutz P, Thierbach A, Geier W (1995) Integrales Konzept Rettungsdienst/Großschadenslage. Notfallmedizin 21:589-592
19. Manji M, Bion JF (1995) Transporting critically ill patients. Intensive Care Med 21:781-783
20. Pearl RG, Mihm FG, Rosenthal MH (1987) Care of the adult patient during transport. Int Anesthesiol Clin 25:43-75
21. Pepe PE, Almaguer DR (1989) Emergency medical services personnel and ground transport vehicles. Prob Crit Care 3:470-476
22. Ridley S, Carter R (1989) The effects of secondary transport on critically ill patients. Anaesthesia 44:822-827
23. Silbergleit R, Dedrick DK, Burney RE, Pape P (1991) Forces acting during transport on patients stabilized by standard immobilisation techniques. Ann Emerg Med 20:875-877
24. Ufer MR (1996) Strukturwandel im Notarztdienst aufgrund höchstrichterlicher Rechtsprechung. Notfallmedizin 22:94-96
25. Valenzuela TD, Criss E, Copass MK, Luna GK, Rice CL (1990) Critical care air transportation of the severely injured: does long distances transport adversely affect survival? Ann Emerg Med 19:169-172
26. Waydhas C, Schneck G, Duswald KH (1995) Deterioration of respiratory function after intra-hospital transport of critically ill surgical patients. Intensive Care Med 21:784-789
27. Wijngaarden M van, Kortbeek J, Lafreniere R, Cunningham R, Joughin E, Yim R (1996) Air ambulance trauma transport: a quality review. J Trauma 26:202-222
28. Witzel K, Hoppe H, Raschka C (1998) Der präklinische Notfalltransport – welche zusätzliche Belastung stellt er für den Patienten dar? Notarzt 14:27-31

Chapter 5

A pre-hospital pharmacological review

G. Trillò, G. Berlot

The mortality for trauma is still dramatically high despite the continuous developments in the organisation of the Emergency Medical Services (EMS), of emergency departments, and the continuous efforts in the research field relating to this matter. A good paper by Trunkey showed a trimodal distribution of deaths from traumatic injury, the first peak being the nonsurvivable injuries, and the second occurring within the first few hours from the event, and that are due mostly to cerebral injury and haemorrhage [1]. Our resuscitative efforts in the pre-hospital setting are focused on reducing this second peak of mortality, and the use of an appropriate pharmacological approach may help us in this task.

Research in trauma

The international literature pertaining to the use of drugs in the management of severe trauma in the pre-hospital setting is varied and often contrasting. This is quite often due to the problems that arise in conducting ethically acceptable double-blind randomised trial studies in this field. Another problem in the evaluation of outcomes from severe pre-hospital trauma is the lack of uniformity in the collection of data. For avoiding such problems a form, similar to the Utstein Style [2] used in cardiac arrest cases, is currently under development. This will lead to better understanding of traumatic outcome data.

Infusions

One of the livelier debates in the scientific community was and still is the use of fluids for trauma resuscitation in the field. The current ATLS procedures agree for the need of gaining access of two large peripheral intravenous (IV) accesses. Some authors have debated about the sometimes long times needed to place the IV lines, with times reported from 1.5 to 12 min [3, 4], showing that delays in initiating a definitive treatment are a contributor to poor pre-hospital care [5].

This is especially true in penetrating trauma, in which the best rescue strategy is probably the "scoop and run" technique, allowing shorter times from the event to the definitive treatment, i.e. the operating room (OR). The question is still open, especially considering that the cannulation manoeuvres can be performed while the patient is already in the ambulance, en route to the hospital [6].

The debate is about "what" kind of infusion to use and the quantity to infuse even livelier. The latter is somewhat unclear from the aforementioned guidelines that state that we must infuse a sufficient volume to restore normal haemodynamic indices [7].

In fact, a review of the volumes infused during transport showed a mean infusion rate between 17 and 47 ml/min [4], basically small and subtherapeutic volumes. A European study of a Helicopter Emergency Medical Service (HEMS), where a trained physician is part of the rescue team, showed higher intensive care admissions and survival rates with a largely more aggressive volume infusion during transport [8].

Controlled hypotension using limited IV fluid administration has now been suggested for the management of a bleeding patient before OR admission. The authors point out that large fluid volumes given before definitive haemostasis may cause clot dislodgement, further bleeding, dilutional coagulopathy and hypothermia [9, 10].

The best strategy is probably to use different approaches in blunt versus penetrating trauma patients. The former may show beneficial effects from aggressive fluid resuscitation, while the latter may benefit from moderate volume resuscitation, keeping the systemic systolic blood pressure somewhat lower. The optimum degree of hypotension is still unknown, although probably a systolic blood pressure of 80 mmHg is adequate to maintain perfusion of vital organs. Please keep in mind that this rule does not apply to patients presenting head injuries, as it will be described later.

Another eternal debate in the scientific community is between the "best" fluid to infuse, with the two main groups equally divided between crystalloid and colloids. A new party is slowing raising voice in the debate, advocating a certain amount of benefits to the so-called "small volume resuscitation" technique, using hypertonic saline.

We will not try to give a definite answer to this problem, since there is no definite, convincing evidence supporting one ot the other. Different strategies will be equally correct for different patient groups and especially in different logistic situations.

Head trauma

Trauma patients with severe head injury usually present a worse prognosis than the group of traumatic injuries as a whole. Recent guidelines published by the "Journal of Neurotrauma" have given us a well-performed meta-analysis of the literature pertaining to this subject. Specifically, many options were offered in the treatment of a severe head injury patient, especially concerning the prevention or limitation of so-called secondary damage.

Basically, the first priority for the head-injured patient is complete and rapid physiologic resuscitation. No specific treatment should be directed at intracranial hypertension in the absence of signs of transtentorial herniation or progressive neurologic deterioration not attributable to extracranial causes [11].

Specifically, hypotension (as defined as systolic blood pressure <90 mmHg), hypoxia (apnoea or cyanosis in the field or a PaO_2 <60 mmHg) must be scrupulously avoided, if possible, or corrected immediately [12]. A mean arterial pressure of more than 90 mmHg should be maintained in an attempt to maintain a cerebral perfusion pressure of more than 70 mmHg.

Although the aforementioned guidelines recommend [13], as a standard, avoiding hyperventilation, this technique may be necessary in the field to treat a patient presenting signs of intracranial hypertension and is therefore given as an option [11].

The use of mannitol, also in the pre-hospital arena, is effective for the control of raised intracranial pressure after severe head injury and is therefore given as an option together with hyperventilation in a patient with clinical signs of transtentorial herniation [14].

The guidelines also offer as a standard, i.e. principles of patient management that reflect a high degree of clinical certainty, that the use of glucocorticoids is not recommended for improving outcome or reducing intracranial pressure in patients with severe head injury [15].

Intubation techniques

It is a well-known fact that a large percentage of all severe head injury patients will suffer severe secondary brain damage due to hypoxia and hypovolemia episodes in the pre-hospital setting. Endotracheal intubation is the only manoeuvre that gives complete and safe airway control. However, no consensus or guidelines exist as to the better procedure to intubate a patient.

The last revision of the ATLS guidelines stresses the fact that the most important factor leading to the decision of placing an endotracheal tube is the skill and experience of the operator [7].

The different techniques may opt for an oral or rhinotracheal intubation, with the use of different combinations of sedative, hypnotic and myorelaxant drugs.

For sedation or induction of anaesthesia the drugs of choice are the ones that are currently in daily use of an experienced anaesthetist. Basically, we may use intravenous induction agents such as thiopental or propofol in a haemodynamically stable patient or ketamine that may be better since it causes less marked cardiovascular effects thus affecting less the intracranial pressure (ICP). A combination of short or longer-acting benzodiazepines together with an opioid such as fentanyl may be a reasonable choice for some particular circumstances.

All these drugs, apart from some particular situations, should be used together with a muscle relaxant, and in this field the most debated drug is succynilcoline. This short-acting, depolarising muscular blockade agent shows at least two of the criteria usually required to a myorelaxant used in the pre-hospital setting, since they have a fast and reliable onset of action and short duration of action [16].

The drawbacks that are advocated by authors who do not consider succynilcoline a drug of choice are possible cardiac arrhythmias, exaggerated hyperkalemic response, increased intraocular pressure, massseter spasm, and possibly malignant hyperthermia.

Although some new short-acting relaxant drugs, such as rocuronium, are now under trial and may be useful in the pre-hospital trauma rescue setting, the risk-benefit ratio will still guarantee the routine use of succynilcoline as the intubation drug of choice.

Spinal cord injury

Although the incidence of spinal cord injury (SCI) is still dramatically high, this particular situation has been extraordinarily resistant to effective treatment. Many authors, in fact, affirm that the prognosis of SCI is made completely at the time of trauma and that no treatment could change it.

The pharmacological approach in the treatment of SCI dates back to 1969 when the use of steroids drugs was proposed as a way to improve neurological recovery.

The advocated use of methyl prednisolone showed no significant improvement in neurological recovery of motor function or pinprick and light touch sensation between two randomised patient groups in a 1984 study [17].

However, the same Authors in a more recent study [18], already widely accepted and being applied world-wide, showed a significant improvement as compared with those given placebo in both motor function and sensation to pinprick if the treatment was established very after trauma.

Since this study, the protocol is still being applied and is one of the few instances in which large doses of a steroid drug are guaranteed in the pre-hospital trauma setting.

Conclusions

This short review has briefly discussed the most commonly used drugs in the trauma patient and focused on the actual debate that involves some of them. As stated before, no definite answer could be given for some of this lively controversies, especially since it is still very difficult to conduct scientific investigation in the pre-hospital trauma arena. The introduction, expected for this year, of a sort of Utstein Style for trauma data Collection will probably give us some deeper insights in the real results of our therapeutic efforts and allow the scientific committee to refine the guidelines and procedures used.

References

1. Trunkey D (1983) Trauma. Sci Am 249:20-27
2. Cummins R, Chamberlain D, Abramson N et al (1991) Recommended guidelines for uniform reporting of data from out-of-hospital cardiac arrest: the Utstein Style. Task Force of the American Heart Association, the European Resuscitation Council, the Heart and Stroke Foundation of Canada, and the Australian Resuscitation Council. Ann Emerg Med 20:861-874

3. Pons P, Moore E, Cusick J (1988) Pre-hospital venous access in an urban paramedic system: a prospective on-scene analysis. J Trauma 28:1460-1463
4. Kaweski S, Sise M, Virgilio R (1990) The effect of pre-hospital fluids on survival in trauma patients. J Trauma 30:1215-1219
5. Maio R, Burney R, Gregor M et al (1996) A study of preventable trauma mortality in rural Michigan. J Trauma 41:83-90
6. Jacobs L, Sinclair A, Beiser A et al (1984) Pre-hospital advanced life support: benefits in trauma. J Trauma 24:8-13
7. American College of Surgeons Committee on Trauma (1993) Advanced trauma life support course for physicians. American College of Surgeons
8. Nardi G, Massarutti D, Muzzi R et al (1994) Impact of emergency medical helicopter service on mortality for trauma in north-east Italy. A regional prospective audit. European Journal of Emergency Medicine 1:69-77
9. Dalton A (1995) Pre-hospital intravenous fluid replacement in trauma: an outmoded concept? J R Soc Med 88:213-216
10. Bickell W, Wall M, Pepe P (1994) Immediate versus delayed fluid resuscitation for hypotensive patients with penetrating torso injuries. N Engl J Med 331:1105-1109
11. The Brain Trauma Foundation, The American Association of Neurological Surgeons, The Joint Section of Neurotrauma and Critical Care (1996) The integration of brain-specific treatments into the initial resuscitation of the severe head injury patient. J Neurotrauma 13:653-659
12. The Brain Trauma Foundation, The American Association of Neurological Surgeons, The Joint Section of Neurotrauma and Critical Care (1996) Resuscitation of blood pressure and oxygenation. J Neurotrauma 13:661-666
13. The Brain Trauma Foundation, The American Association of Neurological Surgeons, The Joint Section of Neurotrauma and Critical Care (1996) The use of hyperventilation in the acute management of severe traumatic brain injury. J Neurotrauma 13:699-703
14. The Brain Trauma Foundation, The American Association of Neurological Surgeons, The Joint Section of Neurotrauma and Critical Care (1996) The use of mannitol in severe head injury. J Neurotrauma 13:705-709
15. The Brain Trauma Foundation, The American Association of Neurological Surgeons, The Joint Section of Neurotrauma and Critical Care (1996) The role of glucocorticoids in the treatmen of severe head injury. J Neurotrauma 13:715-718
16. Murphy-Macabobby M, Marshall WJ, Schneider C et al (1992) Neuromuscular blockade in aeromedical airway management. Ann Emerg Med 21:664-668
17. Bracken MB, Collins WF, Freeman DF et al (1984) Efficacy of methylprednisolone in acute spinal cord injury. JAMA 251:45-52
18. Bracken MB, Shepard MJ, Collins WF et al (1990) A randomized, controlled trial of methylprednisolone or naloxone in the treatment of acute spinal cord injury. Results of the Second National Acute Spinal Cord Injury Study. N Engl J Med 322:1405-1411

Chapter 6

Haemorrhagic shock: pathophysiology and treatment

G.P. Novelli, A. Di Filippo

Shock is a condition of generalized deficit of tissue perfusion. It is defined as haemorrhagic shock (HS) when the deficit is due to a reduction in blood volume caused by acute haemorrhage. The early response to haemorrhage involves both neural and humoral components. The stimuli that can elicit this neuroendocrine response include hypovolaemia, pain, respiratory disturbances, infections, emotional arousal, changes in temperature and changes in blood glucose; the final response might be modified by ethanol, pre-existing diseases, drug withdrawal, age etc.

The immediate response is an adrenergic one with vasoconstriction and reduction of the capacity of the circulatory system. Blood flow to the heart and brain is maintained but arteriolar and capillary blood flow is minimized. Flow to non vital organs is greatly diminished and that to the kidney is reduced to 5%-10% of normal.

Acute hypovolaemia also initiates other endocrine responses: ACTH, glucagon, cortisol, growth hormone and angiotensin II increase; antidiuretic hormone also increases in an attempt to maintain the body's hydration. Hyperglycaemia and increased blood osmolarity tend to shift fluids from the cells and interstitium into the intravascular space to maintain circulating volume.

Diagnostic signs of HS are, normally, easy to identify but, sometimes, they are confused if an external haemorrhage is absent.

Several authors have established clinical categories of haemorrhage based on the volume of blood lost. Loss of 10%-15% of the circulating blood volume (500-750 ml in a 70 kg patient) will cause minimal change in the patient clinical status (class I). A 20%-30% decrease in blood volume will cause the patient to be anxious, mildly tachycardic but a normal arteriolar blood pressure is maintained (class II). With blood volume loss of 30%-40% the classical findings of haemorrhagic shock are apparent (class III). The patient is tachycardic, hypotensive, oliguric or anuric, agitated or confused. Greater than 40% blood loss (>2000 ml in a 70 kg patient) is very severe and the patient may arrive in a moribund condition (class IV). With this degree of blood loss, the patient may become comatose as the blood flow to the brain becomes insufficient to maintain function.

Other precocious signs of haemorrhage or HS are pallor, increased capillary refilling time, clammy and cold skin, fainting, hyperpnoea and tachypnoea with near normal PaO_2 and low $PaCO_2$.

Laboratory data are diminished serum haematocrit and haemoglobin and increased lactate levels.

Haemodynamic data consist of decreased DO_2 and VO_2, low central venous pressure, increased peripheral vascular resistances and decrease cardiac output.

Acute hypovolaemia which is adequately compensated by neuroendocrine responses is termed "compensated".

If HS is so severe that organ and cellular dysfunction occur, the stage of "not compensated" or "progressive shock" develops. This is a critical point because if haemorrhage continues, fluid resuscitation is inadequate, microcirculatory maldistribution is unaffected, and the stage of uncompensated shock (many years ago named "irreversible") develops.

When the haemorrhage is not apparent, the other diagnoses that must be considered include cardiac tamponade, tension pneumothorax, myocardial contusion, myocardial infarction, neurogenic or spinal shock.

The clinical therapeutic goals of severe haemorrhage are: 1) to ensure the vital functions; 2) to ensure adequate intravascular access; 3) to provide adequate quantity and quality of fluids (cristalloids, colloids, blood); and 4) to control of bleeding soruces.

The statements summarized above are very trivial and universally known; the aim of this paper is to report the current state of knowledge of the pathophysiology of HS that concern the following topics:
- ischaemia/hypoxia;
- oxygen reactives intermediates (OR°);
- reperfusion;
- gut ischaemia;
- endothelial changes;
- leucocyte activation;
- NO and peroxynitrite;
- adrenergic receptors.

Ischaemia/hypoxia are basic in the modern appraisal of the pathophysiology of HS as causes of a decrease in cellular level of ATP. The reduction in activity of Na-K, ATP-dependent pump causes an increase in water and sodium intracellular content and consequent cellular swelling [1]. Altered permeability of cell membrane hits calcium channels, too, with an intracellular increase in calcium levels that: 1) stimulate contraction of intracellular skeleton; 2) activate phospholipase with subsequent release of free fatty acids and activation of arachidonic acid cascade; and 3) activate proteolytic processes (such as proteases and endonucleases) which can lead to cell death [2].

Therefore, attempts to inhibit calcium influx in the cells have been made by administration of Ca_{2+} channel blockers [3], SOD [4], and sodium bicarbonate [5]; the results showed that all these drugs obtain a reduction in hepatocyte calcium influx.

Moreover, ischaemia/hypoxia causes profound alterations on the functions of liver, particularly on Kupffer cell (KC) modulation of hepatic function and its response to endotoxin (LPS). In fact ischaemia/hypoxia modify LPS signalling processing by KC that are the major source of IL-6 after haemorrhage [6] and hypoxia [7].

The cytokine IL-1 is released by KC during ischaemia/hypoxia and its production in response to LPS is augmented in this condition [8]. The altered response of KC to LPS during ischaemia/hypoxia is relevant to pathophysiology of HS because the liver (due to its dual blood supply) is submitted firstly to ischaemia/hypoxia from vasoconstriction and secondly to LPS translocating from the ischaemic gut.

Hypoxia alone is sufficient to significantly increase IL-8 gene expression in human endothelial cells [9]. Furthermore, the reduction of cellular oxygen content cause the reduction in ATP levels quoted before and increase in the ratio of NADH/NAD, leading to intracellular acidosis [10].

To improve liver hypoxia during HS some therapeutics was tested.

1. Makisalo et al. found that hydroxyethyl starch and Dextran-70 had the same efficacy to restore liver oxygenation [11] whereas resuscitation with crystalloid fails to improve liver oxygenation in spite of the use of dobutamine [12], probably as a consequence of endothelial oedema induced by crystalloid that reduces tissue oxygen tensions [13].

2. More recently, pentoxifylline was found to improve tissue oxygenation [14] due to its activity on microcirculatory blood flow; although an inhibition of TNF has been claimed [15].

3. Diaspirine cross-linked hemoglobin was recently found to restore peripheral subcutaneous O_2 tension as well as blood but with a longer duration of action [16].

The role of OR° in the pathogenesis of all kinds of shock has been largely discussed by ourselves [17]; such a role is based on global ischaemia-reperfusion during haemorrhage and on activation of granulocyte by cytokines and complement.

PMN appear to have a key role in the pathogenesis of damage consequent to HS; the effector of injury mediated by PMN is the extracellular release of OR° generated by the highly specialized $NADPH:O_2:oxidoreductase$ that has cytosolic and membrane-associated components [18].

SOD inhibits calcium influx in the cells [4] during HS related ischaemia/hypoxia. Furthermore, GSH intracellular level diminishes during ischaemia/reperfusion due to haemorrhage [19] as a defence against OR° overgeneration.

However, a new interesting role for OR° in shock is that one of intracellular signal second messengers. The nuclear transcription regulatory factors are proteins that bind a specific nucleotide sequence in the promoter of genes. One of these is the nuclear factor κB (NFκB) that controls the inducible expression of a variety of genes involved in the immune response (cytokines, cytokine receptors, major histocompatibility complex antigens, acute-phase proteins, and viral enhancers). Schulze-Osthoff et al. [20] reported that mitochondrial-derived ROI functioned as transducers of TNF-induced gene expression being the cofactors of thyrosine protein kinase that catalyses the activation of NFκB [21]. Haemorrhage can induce NFκB action by overproduction of OR° [22] and the redox state of cell and the content of antioxidants as GSH can modify the cellular response to HS [23].

The role of xanthine oxidase (XO) during ischaemia/reperfusion injury is well known in relation to OR° generation. However, Pinault et al. found that immunosuppression during HS in not due to XO action [24] and Mannion et al. affirmed that the benefical effect of XO inhibition with allopurinol on survival may be due to preservation of adenine nucleotides rather than prevention of radical formation [25].

However, the use of antioxidant and OR° scavengers protects and ameliorates ischaemia reperfusion injury induced by XO OR° overproduction in several models, particularly in the gut [26]. Leucocyte adhesion has been implicated as a critical step in vascular endothelium injury, leading to increased microvascular permeability and thrombosis with flow difficulty at reperfusion [27].

Intestinal damage is mostly damage to the intestinal villus submitted to blood flow reduction. In this case there is a passage of oxygen content from the basal arteriolar blood supply to the venous circle in the basal part of the villus and consequent ischaemia of the apex of the vill. This can be prevented by administration of allopurinol [28] or SOD [29].

Apical ischaemia of the villus can cause translocation of endotoxin and bacteria activating the complement cascade of liver KC to release TNF; in fact, germ free rats are more tolerant to HS than the germ bearing ones [30].

Some controversy does exist about gut translocation and its role in HS. Moore et al. were unable to document the presence of bacteria or endotoxin in the portal or systemic blood of trauma victims [31] and, also, the selective decontamination of the digestive tract of ICU patients did not improve survival [32].

Trauma and HS-associated intestinal ischaemia and loss of intestinal barrier function results in exposure to bacteria and/or their products of the gut-associated lymphatic tissue (GALT) [33]. GALT contains 50% of the lymphoid cells of the body and its activation provokes a very large release of cytokines during HS [34].

Endothelial changes affect coagulation balance, regulation of vasomotor tone, vascular permeability and leucocyte adhesion and activation. In the setting of ischaemia/reperfusion but more importantly in inflammation injury, the endothelium is shifted to a prothrombotic state both by inhibition of anticoagulant pathways and enhancement of procoagulant factors [35]. Regulation of vascular tone and leukocyte response are depicted below. The vascular permeability is altered by a direct toxic effect on endothelial cells of OR° [36]. The mechanism of damage seems to be endothelial cell apoptosis induction that is prevented by antioxidant administration [37]. IL-8 gene expression in human endothelial cells significantly increases after exposition to ischemia/hypoxia [9].

Leucocytes are activated by cytokines and endotoxin and are the main site of production of OR°.

Another field of interest in HS is the induction, by hypoxia, ischaemia and reperfusion complex cell response, of altered interaction through endothelial cells and circulating leucocytes [38].

These interactions are mediated by numerous adhesion molecules that can be divided into three families: the selectins, the integrins, and the immunoglobulin supergene family [39].

The interaction between these molecules takes place in three steps [35]: an initial step is mediated by loose associations between E and P selectins (i.e. ELAM-1) expressed by activated endothelial cells and L-selectins (on surface of PMN). Then the PMN begin to roll on the surface of the endothelium and the integrins CD11a, b and c/CD18 of the leucocyte surface interact with ICAM 1 and 2 of the endothelial cells to obtain a firm adhesion between the cells. The final step consists in the migration of PMN through endothelial cells in a process mediated by PECAM-1.

Each step is inducted by the presence of chemotactic agents (the first by IL-8 and LTB4, the second by PAF and IL-8, the last by a chemotactic gradient between the intravascular and extravascular ambient) [35].

Experimental studies using monoclonal antibodies directed against adhesion molecules (principally ICAM-1 and CD11/CD18) showed promising results in various ischaemia/reperfusion rat model [40].

The development of soluble forms of adhesion molecules to compete for ligands is another therapeutic strategy actually under study [41].

Partrick et al., in agreement with the "two hit model" of clinical events during MODS, supposed that the evolution of PMN damage of tissues requires two events: 1) the initial activation that enhances the superoxide anion production and the interactions with endothelium; and 2) the priming that promote further PMN sequestration in the tissue and release of OR° [42].

The principal primer of PMN activation is supposed to be PAF. So, PAF antagonists are proposed as prevention of PMN priming after trauma [43].

More recently the role of PMN in inflammatory response to HS has been discussed: these cells appear to be implicated in the downregulation of cytokine production [44].

The biosynthesis of NO has been discussed mostly as related to sepsis but many data also concern HS [45]. In the initial phases of HS, in fact, there is an impairment of NO synthesis by ecNOS also in cerebral and renal vascular beds that is responsible for reduction of flow in these districts.

Furthermore, since NO is an inhibitor of the adhesion of PMN to the endothelium [46] the reduction of NO production can cause flow impairment by PMN adherence. In fact, infusion of NO donors reduces the degree of PMN infiltration and prevents endothelial dysfunction [47].

After words (48-72 h) a progressive fall in blood pressure occurs due to the progressive vasodilatation (vascular decompensation of the late phase of HS) due to enhanced NO formation by iNOS, as demonstrated by its inhibition with L-NAME and prevention with dexamethasone [48]. INOS can be induced by TNF and IL-1 [49] and PAF [50].

The WEB 2086, a PAF antagonist, partially protects against the impairment of endothelium-dependent relaxation [51]. Finally, NO derived by ecNOS and iNOS, may well contribute to myocardial depression in HS [52].

In front of the numerous side effects of drugs that have modified the bioavailability of NO in the past, different strategies of therapy were produced such as: 1) "selective targeting" of tissue/organ of specific NOS isoenzymes; 2) inhalation therapy with NO gas [53]; 3) lower doses of NO donors; and 4) simultaneous administration of NO donors and NOS inhibitors [54].

Harbrecht et al. reported that inhibition of NO synthetase during HS increases HS-induced hepatic injury at a dose that dit not affect systemic blood pressure because NO prevents leucocyte and platelet accumulation in the hepatic circulation [55].

More recently Kilbourne et al. in a review article of experimental and clinical studies on the effects of NOS inhibition affirmed that a combination of therapeutic approaches that treat not only vasodilatation, but also metabolic dysfunction, coagulation abnormality and multiorgan damage can treat septic shock [56].

One by-product of ROI overproduction, particularly of superoxide and NO overgeneration during HS, is the *peroxynitrite*; the principal effect of this compound is the initiation of DNA strand breakage, which is an obligatory stimulus for the activation of the nuclear enzyme polyADP ribosyl synthetase (PARS); this pathway leads to cell necrosis or apoptosis in HS, as in neurodegenerative disorders, diabetes, stroke etc. [57].

The isothiourea-derived compound mercaptoethylguanidine possesses properties of prevention of the increase in NO and of peroxynitrite scavenging and reduces the suppression of mitochondrial respiration and the development of DNA single-strand breaks [58].

It is increasingly being recognized that the inflammatory immune response during sepsis can be modulated by catecholamines as well as administration of drugs that act on α receptors, particularly $\alpha2$, β and dopaminergic receptors, possibly through changes in cAMP metabolism [59].

$\alpha2$-Adrenergic agonists augment LPS-induced TNF production and this effect is prevented by the antagonist yohimbine [60]; epinephrine increases IL-6 production in both isolated perfused rat liver and isolated KC, mediated via the β-receptor pathway [61]. So, vasopressor and inotropic support of HS can have consequences on the efficacy of immunotherapy.

References

1. Waxman K (1996) Shock: ischemia, reperfusion and inflammation. New Horizons 4:153-160
2. Trump BF, Berezesky IK (1995) Calcium-mediated cell injury and cell death. FASEB J 9:219-218
3. Rose S, Pizanis A, Silomon M (1997) Altered hepato-cellular Ca_{2+} regulation during haemorrhagic shock and resuscitation. Hepatology 25:379-384
4. Rose S, Sayed MM (1997) Superoxide radicals scavenging prevents cellular calcium dysregulation during intrabdominal sepsis. Shock 7:263-268
5. Silomon M, Rose S (1998) Effect of sodium bicarbonate infusion on hepatocyte Ca_{2+} overload during resuscitation from haemorrhagic shock. Resuscitation 37:27-32
6. O'Neil P, Ayala A, Wang P, Ba ZF, Morrison MH, Schultze AE et al (1994) Role of Kupffer cells in IL-6 release following trauma-hemorrage and resuscitation. Shock 1:43-47
7. West MA, Wilson C (1996) Hypoxic alterations in cellular signal transduction in shock and sepsis. New Horizons 2:168-175
8. West MA, Li MH, Seatter SC et al (1994) Pre-exposure to hipoxia and septic stimuli differentially regulates endotoxin release of TNF, IL-6, IL-1, PGE2, NO, and superoxide by macrophages. J Trauma 37:82-90
9. Karukurum M, Shreeniwas R, Chen J et al (1994) Hypoxic induction of IL-8 gene expression in human endothelial cells. J Clin Invest 93:1564-1570
10. Gores G, Nieminen A, Wray B (1989) Intracellular pH during chemical hypoxia in coultured rats hepatocytes. J Clin Invest 83:386-396
11. Makisalo HJ, Soini HO, Tapani Lalla ML et al (1988) Subcutaneous and liver tissue oxygen tension in haemorrhagic shock: and experimental study with whole blood and two colloids. Crit Care Med 16:857-861

12. Nordin AJ, Makisalo H, Hockerstedt KAV (1996) Failure of dobutamine to improve liver oxygenation during resuscitation with crystalloid solution after experimental haemorrhagic shock. Eur J Surg 162:973-979
13. Heughan C, Niinikoski J, Hunt TK (1972) Effect of excessive infusion of saline solution on tissue oxygen transport. Surg Gynecol Obstet 135:257-260
14. Waxman K, ClarK L, Soliman MH, Parizin S (1991) Pentoxifylline in resuscitation of experimental hemmorrhagic shock. Crit Care Med 19:728-731
15. Lilly CM, Sandhu S, Ishizaka A et al (1989) Pentoxifylline prevents TNF-induced lung injury. Am Rev Resp Dis 139:1361-1368
16. Powell CC, Schultz SC, Burris DG et al (1995) Subcutaneous oxygen tension: a useful adjunct in assessment of perfusion status. Crit Care Med 23:867-873
17. Novelli GP (1997) Role of free radicals in septic shock. J Physiol Pharmacol 48:517-527
18. Clarck RA (1990) The Human neutrophil respiratory burst oxidase. J Infect Dis 161:1140-1147
19. Reuter A, Klinger W (1992) The influence of systemic hypoxia and reoxigenation on the glutathione redox system of brain, liver, lung and plasma of newborn rats. Exp Toxicol Pathol 44:339-343
20. Schulze-Osthoff K, Beyeart R, Vandevoorde V (1993) Depletion of the mitochondrial electron transporte abrogates the cytotoxic and gene-inductive effects of TNF. EMBO J 12:3095-3104
21. Suzuki YJ, Mizuno M, Packer L (1994) Signal transduction for NFK B activation: proposed location for antioxidant inhibitable step. J Immunol 153:5008-5015
22. Abraham E (1996) Alterations in transcriptional regulation of proinflammatory and immunoregulatory cytokine expression by haemorrhage, injury and critical illness. New Horizons 2:184-191
23. Staal FJ, Anderson MT, Staal GEJ et al (1994) Redox regulation of signal transduction: tyrosine phosphorylation and calcium influx. Proc Natl Acad Sci USA 91:619-623
24. Pinault GC, Sanson AJ, Malangoni MA (1997) Inhibition of xanthine oxidase does not influence immunosuppression after haemorrhagic shock. J Trauma 43:911-915
25. Mannion D, Fitzpatrick GJ, Feeley M (1994) Role of xanthine oxidase inhibition in survival from haemorrhagic shock. Circ Shock 42:39-43
26. Schoemberg MH, Muhl E, Sellin D (1984) Posthypotensive generation of superoxide free radicals possible role in the pathogenesis of intestinal mucosa damage. Acta Chir Scand 150:301-309
27. Ar'Rajab A, Dawidson I, Fabia R (1996) Reperfusion injury. New Horizons 4:224-234
28. Deitch EA, Bridges W, Baker J et al (1988) Haemorrhagic shock induced bacterial translocation is reduced by xanthine oxidase inhibition or inactivation. Surgery 104:191-198
29. Novelli GP, Livi P, Falsini S et al (1989) Prevenzione del danno da riperfusione mesenterica nel coniglio mediante antiossidanti. Acta Anesth Italica 40:345-355
30. Ferraro FJ, Rush BF, Simonian GT et al (1995) A comparison of survival at different degrees of haemorrhagic shock in germ free and germ bearing rats. Shock 4:117-120
31. Moore FA, Moore EA, Poggetti R (1991) Gut bacterial traslocation via the portal vein: a clinical perspective with major torso trauma. J Trauma 31:629-638
32. Van Saene HKF, Stoutenbeek CC, Stoller JK (1992) Selective decontamination of digestive tract in ICU: current status and future prospects. Crit Care Med 20:691-703
33. Deitch EA, Rutan R, Waymack JP (1996) Trauma, shock and gut traslocation. New Horizons 4:289-299
34. Deitch EA, Xu D, Franko L et al (1994) Evidence favouring the role of the gut as a cytokine-generating organ in rats subjected to Haemorrhagic shock. Shock 1:141-146

35. Maier RV, Bulger EM (1996) Endothelial changes after shock and injury. New Horizons 4:211-223
36. Ratych R, Chuknyiska R, Bulkley G (1987) The primary localization of free radicals generation after after anoxia/reoxygenation in isolated endothelial cells. Surgery 102:122-131
37. Abello P, Fidler S, Bulkley G (1994) Antioxidant modulate induction of programmed endothelial cell death by endotoxin. Arch Surg 129:134-141
38. Scannell G (1996) Leukocyte responses to hypoxic/ischemic conditions. New Horizons 4:179-183
39. Abelda S, Smith C, Ward P (1994) Adhesion molecules and inflammatory injury. FASEB J 8:504-512
40. Mileski W, Winn R, Vedder N (1990) Inhibition of CD18 dependent PMN adherence reduces organ injury after haemorrhagic shock in primates. Surgery 108:206-212
41. Gamble J, Skinner M, Berndt M (1990) Prevention of activated neutrophil adhesion to endothelium by soluble adhesion protein GMP 140. Science 249:414-417
42. Partrick DA, Moore FA, Moore EE, Barnett CC et al (1996) Neutrophil priming and activation in the pathogenesis of post-injury MOF. New Horizons 4:194-210
43. Heuer HO, Casals-Stenzel J, Muacevic G et al (1990) Pharmacologic activity of bepafant [WEB 2170], a new selective hetrazapinoic antagonist of PAF. J Pharmacol Exp Ther 255:962-968
44. Omert L, Tsukada K, Hierholzer C et al (1998) A role of neutrophils in the down regulation of IL-6 and CD14 following haemorrhagic shock. Shock 6:391-396
45. Szabò C, Thiemermann C (1993) Invited opinion: role of NO in haemorrhagic, traumatic and anaphylactic shock and thermal injury. Shock 2:145-155
46. Gabury J, Woodman RC, Granger DN (1993) NO prevents Leukocyte adherence: role of superoxide. Am J Physiol 265:H862-H867
47. Symington PA, Ma XL, Lefer AM (1992) Protective actions of S-nitrtoso-Nacetylpenicillamine - SNAP - in a rat model of haemorrhagic shock. Methods Find Exp Clin Pharmacol 14:789-797
48. Thiemermann C, Szabò C, Mitchell JA, Vane JR (1993) Vascular hyporeactivity to vasoconstrictor agents and haemodynamic decompensation in haemorrhagic shock mediated by NO. Proc Natl Acad Sci USA 90:267-271
49. Kilbourne RG, Gross SS, Jubran A, Adams J et al (1990) N-methyl-L-Arginine inhibits TNF induced hypotension: implications for the involvment of NO. Proc Natl Acad Sci USA 87:3629-3632
50. Szabò C, Mitchell JA, Gross SS et al (1993) PAF contributes to the induction of NO synthetase by bacterial lipopolysaccharide. Circ Res 73:991-999
51. Csaki C, Szabò C, Kovac AGB (1992) Role of PAF in the development of endothelial dysfunction in haemorrhagic hypotension and retrasfusion. Thrombosis Res 66:23-31
52. Brady AJB, Poole-Wilson PA, Harding SE et al (1992) NO production within cardiac myocytes reduces their contractility in endotoxemia. Am J Physiol 263:H1963-H1966
53. Weizberg E, Rudehill A, Lundberg JM (1993) NO inhalation attenuates hypertension and improves gas exchanges in endotoxin shock. Eur J Pharmacol 233:85-94
54. Wright CE, Rees DD, Moncada S (1992) Protective and pathological roles of NO in endotoxin shock. Cardiovasc Res 26:48-57
55. Harbrecht BG, Wu B, Watkins SC et al (1995) Inhibition of NOS during haemorrhagic shock increases hepatic injury. Shock 4:332-337
56. Kilbourne RG, Szabò C, Traber DL (1997) Benefical versus detrimental effects of NO synthase inhibitors in circulatory shock: lesson learned from experimental and clinical studies. Shock 7:235-246

57. Szabò C (1996) DNA Strand breakage and activation of PARS a cytotoxic pathway triggered by peroxynitrite. Free Rad Biol and Med 21:855-869
58. Zingarelli B, Ischiropulos HI, Salzman AL et al (1997) Amelioration by mercaptoethylguanidine of the vascular and energetic failure in haemorrhagic shock in anesthetised rat. Eur J Pharmacol 338:55-65
59. Pastores McCarthy S, Hasko G, Vizi S et al (1996) Cytokine production and its manipulation by vasoactive drugs. New Horizons 4:252-264
60. Spengler RN, Allen RM, Remick DG (1990) Stimulation of adrenergic receptor augments of macrophage derived TNF. J Immunol 145:1430-1445
61. Liao J, Keiser JA, Scales WE et al (1995) Role of epinephrine in TNF and IL-6 production from isolated perfused rat liver. Am J Physiol 268:R896-R901

Chapter 7

Fluid management in trauma

J. BOLDT

Trauma-related hypovolemia may be associated with flow alterations which are inadequate to fulfill the nutritive role of the circulation [1]. During this hypovolemia-related low output syndrome (LOS), the organism tries to compensate perfusion deficits by redistribution of flow to vital organs (i.e., heart and brain) resulting in an underperfusion of other organs such as splanchnic bed, kidney, muscles, and skin. Various inflammatory mediators and circulating vasoactive substances are of particular importance for impaired perfusion in trauma patients. Activation of the sympathetic nervous system and the renin-angiotensin system (RAS) are compensatory mechanisms to maintain peripheral perfusion. Although this compensatory neurohumoral activation is beneficial at first, this mechanism becomes deleterious and may be involved in the poor outcome of the critically ill [2].

The risk of transmission of viral diseases has forced us to reduce the use of allogeneic blood to restore volume deficits. Reduction in hematocrit and in arterial oxygen content is not deleterious since compensating mechanisms are able to guarantee tissue oxygenation and systemic oxygen transport. Myocardial oxygen supply is determined by coronary blood flow and its oxygen content. Augmentation of coronary blood flow may not provide adequate myocardial oxygenation when arterial blood oxygen content is decreased by reducing hemoglobin levels due to (extreme) hemodilution. When non-blood volume is used to replace volume deficits, the margin of safety may become compromised especially in patients with significant coronary obstruction: there is an increasing risk of a discrepancy between myocardial oxygen requirements and available subendocardial oxygen supply, which may result in the deterioration of myocardial performance.

Another important aspect of fluid therapy in the traumatized patient is the risk of inducing interstitial edema. Tissue edema is related to an imbalance in the sum of the Starling forces across capillary membranes or an increase in protein permeability, by which an increase in fluid flux in the interstitial space is promoted. A decrease in membrane integrity, an increase in hydrostatic pressure, and a decrease in intravascular colloid oncotic pressure (COP) will induce fluid movement across the microvascular membrane and may produce interstitial fluid accumulation.

Adequate volume therapy is a mainstay for treating trauma patients. The controversy in this area focuses on the ideal kind of volume therapy [3-7]. Besides human albumin (HA) and crystalloids, synthetic colloids such as gelatins, dextrans or hydroxethylstarch (HES) solution are often used. The current tendency in Europe is to infuse colloid solutions rather than large amounts of Ringer's solution for volume replacement. Dextran may be associated with severe anaphlyactic reactions and marked deterioration in coagulation. HES solution is becoming very popular and is the most widespread solution for volume therapy in several countries. "Optimal" volume replacement in trauma patients, however, is still discussed controversially.

Strategies to restore volume deficits

Crystalloids are widely used for restoration of volume deficits in the USA. Crystalloids do not vary significantly among the different preparations. They are freely permeable to the vascular membrane and are therefore distributed in the plasma and interstitial fluid volume. After 1 000 ml saline infusion, plasma volume was expanded by only 180 ml [8]. Thus large volumes of crystalloids are required for restoring sufficient hemodynamics after bleeding (i.e. compensation of 1 000 ml blood loss requires approximately 3 000-4 000 ml crystalloids). When infusing such hugh quantities of unbuffered saline, hyperchloremic acidosis could theoretically complicate this kind of volume therapy. Dilution of plasma protein concentration may also follow, resulting in a reduction in COP subsequently leading to tissue edema.

Colloids have to be separated into natural colloids (human albumin preparations) and synthetic colloids (different preparations of gelatins, HES, and dextrans). Albumin is a naturally occurring plasma protein and, in spite of its high cost, it is still widely used in many institutions. The molecular weight of albumin ranges from 66 000 to 69 000 daltons. Due to its method of preparation, it is free of risk of transmitting infections. A 5% albumin solution is iso-oncotic, whereas 20% and 25% solutions are markedly hyperoncotic, so that total plasma volume is expanded by translocation of fluid from the interstitial to the intravascular compartment. The effects of 5% albumin are not readily predictable: infusion of 500 ml albumin expanded plasma volume by 490 ml or 750 ml. The retention of the infused albumin in the intravascular compartment and therefore its hemodynamic efficacy greatly varies depending on the patient's disease. In patients with altered vascular endothelial integrity, albumin may pass into the interstitial space, by which fluid shift from the intravascular compartment may be promoted. The importance of albumin is also related to its transport function for various drugs and endogenous substances (i.e., bilirubin, free fatty acids).

Many drugs used in the critically ill bind to albumin, and drug toxicity is partly attributable to altered binding capacity. Last but not least, antioxidant properties of albumin have been described [9]. Synthetic colloids are more and more often used for volume replacement due to cost containment strategies. Gelatin exists in two major modifications: modified fluid gelatin and urea-bridged gelatin. The only major differences between these preparations are different electrolyte concentrations. The increase in blood volume is approximately the same as that of the infused volume of gelatin (range 70%-90%). However, due to the low molecular weight average (approximately 35 000), the plasma half-life is only short (1-2.0 h) so that early re-infusion is necessary to maintain adequate blood volume. The incidence of severe anaphylactic reaction mediated by histamine liberation has been significantly lowered by reducing the amount of cross-linked agents but appears to be still a problem when using gelatins [10]. Dextrans are linear polysaccharide molecules of high molecular weight. Two different preparations are available: 6% dextran 70 (average molecular weight 70 000 daltons) and 10% dextran 40 (average molecular weight 40 000 daltons). Increases in plasma volume after infusion of 1 000 ml of dextran 70 ranged from 600 to 800 ml. The main differences between these two solutions concern their influence on microcirculation. Infusion of dextran 40 increases microcirculatory flow because of reduced red cell and platelet sludging, volume expansion, and hemodilution-induced reduction in whole blood viscosity. Different preparations of HES solutions are available with different concentrations (3%, 6%, 10%), different molecular weight averages (MW) (70 000 daltons, low MW; 200 000-270 000 daltons, medium MW; 450 000 daltons, high MW) and different degrees of molar substitution ratio (MS) (0.5, 0.62, 0.7). The extent and duration of plasma expansion are extremely dependent on the physical and chemical characteristics of HES solution. Thus maintenance of hemodynamic stability seems to be highly dependent on the kind of HES preparation used. Depending on the HES preparation, different effects on rheology, coagulation, oncotic pressure, and intravascular half-lives are observed [11, 12].

Trauma and organ hypoperfusion

Severe trauma is often associated with hypoperfusion of various organ systems. Circulatory abnormalities may be caused by an excessive or inadequate humoral neuroendocrine response. Trauma may result in adrenocortical stimulation and activation of the sympathetic system leading to the release of an array of hormones which are responsible for the regulation of organ perfusion. Recent evidence suggests that the endothelium is not only a passive barrier between the circulating blood and the tissue, but may also be markedly involved in the regulation of microcirculatory blood flow by producing important regulators of vascular tone, i.e., prostaglandins, nitric oxide (NO), endothelins, angiotensin II [13, 14]. Thus the regional regulation of blood flow is likely due to a balance between systemic (central) mechanisms (i.e., the autononous nervous system) and other circulating or locally active blood flow regulators. One important approach to improve perfusion in the critically ill is the use of sufficient volume replacement. There is controversy in this area as to which kind of solution is best in avoiding the sequelae of trauma-related volume deficits. Unfortunately, most studies only compared short-term effects of volume infusion [3], and definite evaluation of the efficacy of the various volume replacement regimes is not possible with this study design. In a prospective randomized study long-term volume therapy using either HES (10%, 200/0.5) or 20% HA was studied in trauma patients showing an injury severity score (ISS) <15 points [15]. HA or HES was exclusively infused over 5 days to keep pulmonary capillary wedge pressure (PCWP) between 10 and 15 mmHg. Besides hemodynamic monitoring, liver function was assessed using a monoethylglycinexylidide (MEGX) test, and gastric intramucosal pH (pHi) was monitored by tonometry to evaluate splanchnic perfusion. Additionaly, important circulatory regulators were measured from arterial blood samples (i.e., vasopressin, endothelin-1, epinephrine, norepinephrine, atrial natriuretic peptide, 6-keto-prostaglandin $F_{1\alpha}$). Mean arterial pressure (MAP), heart rate (HR), and PCWP did not differ between the two groups. Cardiac index (CI) increased significantly more in the HES than in the HA groups. pHi and MEGX plasma levels were without differences in the trauma patients throughout the study period. Concentrations of all vasoactive regulators showed an almost similar course in both volume groups. It was concluded that, in trauma patients, long-term volume therapy with albumin or HES solution did not differ with regard to changes in important macro- and microcirculatory regulators. Liver function and perfusion in the splanchnic bed were also without differences between HA- and HES-treated trauma patients. Thus synthetic volume replacment using HES 200/0.5 can be safely used in these patients, while the still widespread use of HA for volume therapy cannot be recommended in trauma patients.

Trauma, volume replacement and coagulation

Documented and theoretical hazards are associated with all fluids used for volume replacement. Trauma patients often show a wide spectrum of coagulation abnormalities. This may result in an imbalance between the procoagulant and inhibitory activities of the coagulation system. Further alterations in coagulation should be avoided when choosing the "ideal" volume replacement strategy. Although there seems to be no convincing clinical advantage, HA is still widely used in several centers to treat patients with increased bleeding risk [16]. There is concern that some synthetic colloids may have an adverse effect on coagulation. Dextran, i.e., is known to be associated with severe deterioration in coagulation with subsequent increased bleeding. Macromolecules are assumed to coat the outer membrane of circulating platelets, thus causing a qualitative platelet function defect. The mechanisms by which synthetic colloids exert their platelet inhibiting effects have not been fully elucidated. When using dextran, both VIIIR:Ag and VIIIR:RCo levels decrease significantly. With reduced VIIIR:RCo there is reduced binding to platelet membrane receptor proteins GPIb and GPIIb/IIIa, which results in a decreased platelet adhesion. Gelatins are also often used for volume replacement in trauma patients because it is assumed that volume therapy with gelatins is associated with less bleeding problems. The effects of gelatins on hemostasis were recently studied by de Jonge in healthy humans receiving either 1 000 ml gelatin or saline solution [17]. Infusion of gelatin resulted in significant impairment of primary hemostasis and thrombin generation. The defect in primary hemostasis appears to be related to a gelatin-induced reduction in von Willbrand factor. The authors concluded that gelatins should be given cautiously to patients with preexisting abnormal platelet function, and massive transfusions with gelatins should be avoided.

The effects of the various preparations of HES on the coagulation process have only been partially defined. Both normal and abnormal platelet aggregation were reported. High molecular weight (HMW)-HES diminished the concentrations of VIIIR:Ag and VIIIR:RCo more pronouncedly than lower molecular weight (LMW)-HES. After large doses of HMW-HES, platelets appeared swollen, and platelet adhesion was reduced. LMW-HES (MW 270 000 daltons; pentastarch) was reported to have overall fewer negative effects on the coagulation system [18-20]. In a study in cardiac surgery patients, it was shown that, overall HMW-HES resulted in the most pronounced impairment of platelet aggregation and thus it should be avoided in patients with an increased risk of higher postoperative bleeding [21]. LMW-HES did not show the same negative effects on platelet aggregation as were seen in the HMW-HES group. It is of particular importance that albumin, which is favoured in many centers, did not differ from LMW-HES- and gelatin-treated patients with regard to platelet function, post-bypass bleeding, and the need for homologous blood. These results provide reasons to question the use/abuse of albumin in patients at bleeding risk.

Most studies reporting on increased bleeding tendency with HES used HMW (450 000 daltons) high-substituted (0.7) HES (i.e., hetastarch in the USA) [22]. Modern HES solutions with lower molecular weight (70 000 or 200 000 daltons) and which are lower substituted (0.5) yield significantly less alterations in coagulation and can thus be safely used also in the bleeding trauma patient. A new HES preparation (130 000/0.4) that will be available in several countries in the near future appears to be associated with even less alterations in the hemostatic network.

Trauma, volume replacement and the immune system

Traumatic injury is known to induce alterations of cell-mediated and humoral immunity [23-25]. This sequelae of trauma predispose the patient to the development of sepsis or systemic inflammatory response syndrome (SIRS). The mediators of immunosuppression secondary to trauma have not been definitively elucidated. Endotoxin, tissue metabolic products resulting from cellular hypoxia, shock proteins, and hormonal mediators (i.e., catecholamines) are suspected to take part in this complex process of immunmodulation. Polymorphonuclear cells (PMNs) are thought supposed to be key mediators of tissue injury and organ failure in trauma patients [26]. While neutrophils are essential for bacterial killing, they paradoxically have the capacity to injure host tissue. The accumulation of activated neutrophils appears to play a key role in the pathogenesis of SIRS and development of multiple organ failure (MOF). The interactions of neutrophils with endothelial cells are regulated by complementary adhesion molecules, which are expressed by these cells. Three different main groups of adhesion molecules can be distinguished [27, 28]: 1) the immunoglobulin superfamily (IGSF), i.e., vascular cell adhesion molecule-1 (VCAM-1); intercellular adhesion molecule-1 (ICAM-1); 2) the integrin family, i.e., lymphocyte function-associated antigen (LFA-1=CD11a/CD18); and 3) the selectins, E-selectin (endothelial leukocyte adhesion molecule, ELAM-1), L-selectin (i.e., leukocyte endothelial cell adhesion molecule, LECAM), and P-selectin (granule membrane protein 140, GMP-140).

Soluble forms of some adhesion molecules have been identified in the circulating blood [29, 30]. They appear to be excellent markers of inflammation, endothelial activation or damage [31]. The influence of different volume replacement strategies on circulating adhesion molecules has been studied in a prospective randomized study using either human albumin (20% HA) or HES (10% HES 200/0.5) in 30 trauma patients showing an ISS >15 points [32]. Volume was given over 5 days to keep central venous pressure (CVP) and/or PCWP between 12 and 18 mm Hg. At baseline, plasma levels of all measured adhesion molecules were similar in both groups. In the HES patients, sELAM-1 and sICAM-1 plasma levels decreased significantly reaching normal values within the study period, whereas they increased in the HA-group (sICAM-1: from 400±81 to 749±101 ng/ml). sVCAM-1 increased beyond normal range only in the HA-group (to 760±69 ng/ml). sGMP-140 plasma concentration increased only in the HA-patients (from 432±85 to 550±93 ng/ml). It was concluded that an increased knowledge of immunology and molecular biology have broadened our understanding of the inflammatory consequences in severely traumatized patients. Treatment of these patients should be focused on limiting endothelial activation and damage since this appears to be the initial trigger of the development of multiple organ deficiency syndrome (MODS). In comparison to HA, infusion of HES resulted in a reduction in circulating adhesion molecules indicating unimproved endothelial function in HES-treated trauma patients.

In summary volume replacement is known to be a therapeutic cornerstone in treating the trauma patient. Guarantee or restoration of tissue perfusion represents a particular challenge in patients with circulatory abnormalities. The efficacy of different fluid preparations in this situation is still controversial. Replenishment of intravascular volume cannot always sufficiently prevent the deleterious consequences of abnormalities in microcirculation and nutritive tissue flow. Blood volume can be definitely restored more rapidly with colloid solutions. Even excessive amounts of crystalloids do not always guarantee circulating blood volume and sufficient hemodynamics. In spite of an immense amount of information regarding this problem, there is still no solution. In recent years the crystalloid-colloid debate has been extended by a colloid-colloid debate. When comparing albumin and synthetic colloids, there are several studies that have demonstrated no differences between these colloids. The physiological effect, namely sufficient stabilization of circulation, that is achieved appears to be more important than the agent used to achieve this effect. The ideal solution should not only maintain gross hemodynamics, but microcirculation should also be guaranteed, or even improved, without being associated with significant side effects. Financial considerations may, legitamately, come increasingly into play. The major advantage of synthetic colloids compared to albumin is their relative low cost. Long-term volume therapy with albumin appears to be without benefit for the critically ill. Infusion of LMW-HES is an attractive alternative which may result in significantly better systemic hemodynamics and organ perfusion than volume replacement with HA.

References

1. Intaglietta M (1990) Objectives for the treatment of the microcirculation in ischemia, shock, and reperfusion. In: Vincent JL (ed) Update in intensive care and emergency medicine. Vol 10. Springer-Verlag, Berlin Heidelberg New York, pp 293-298
2. Turnbull AV, Little RA (1993) Neuro-hormonal regulation after trauma. Circulating cytokines may also contribute to an activated sympathetic-adrenal control. In: Vincent JL (ed) Update in intensive care and emergency medicine. Springer-Verlag, Berlin Heidelberg New York Tokyo, pp 574-581
3. Beards SC, Watt T, Edwards JD et al (1994) Comparison of the hemodynamic and oxygen transport responses to modified fluid gelatin and hetastarch in critically ill patients: a prospective, randomized trial. Crit Care Med 22:600-605
4. Davidson I (1989) Fluid resuscitation of shock: current controversies. Crit Care Med 17:1078-1080
5. Edwards JD, Nightingale P, Wilkins RG et al (1988) Hemodynamic and oxygen transport response to modified fluid gelatin in the critically ill patients. Crit Care Med 17:996-998
6. Prough DS, Johnston WE (1989) Fluid restoration in septic shock: no solution yet. Anesth Analg 69:699-704
7. Vincent JL (1991) The colloid-crystalloid controvery. Klin Wochensch 69(Suppl 26): 104-111
8. Lamke LO, Liljedahl SO (1976) Plasma volume changes after infusion of various plasma expanders. Resuscitation 5:93-98
9. Emmerson TE (1989) Unique features of albumin: a brief review. Crit Care Med 17:690-693
10. Laxenaire M, Charpentier C, Feldman L (1994) Reactions anaphylactoides aux subitutes colloidaux du plasma: incidence, facteurs de risque, mecanismes. Ann Fr Anest Reanim 13:301-310
11. London MJ, Ho SJ, Triedman JK et al (1989) A randomized clinical trial of 10% pentastarch (low molecular weight hydroxyethyl starch) versus 5% albumin for plasma volume expansion after cardiac operations. J Thorac Cardiovasc Surg 97:785-797
12. Webb AR, Barclay SA, Bennett ED (1989) In vitro colloid osmotic pressure of commonly used plasma substitutes: a study of the diffusibility of colloid molecules. Intensive Care Med 15:116-120
13. Brenner BM, Troy JL, Ballermann B (1989) Endothelium-dependent vascular responses. J Clinical Invest 84:1373-1378
14. Lewis DH (1988) The effect of multiple organ failure on the regulation of the circulation with special reference to the microcirculation. In: Manabe H, Zweifach BW, Messmer K (eds) Microcirculation in Circulatory Disorders. Springer-Verlag, Tokyo Berlin Heidelberg, pp 103-108
15. Boldt J, Müller M, Mentges D et al (1996) Influence of different volume therapy regime on regulators of circulation in the critically ill. Br J Anaesth 77:480-487
16. Boldt J, Lenz M, Kumle B et al (1998) Volume replacement strategies on intensive care units: results from a postal survey. Intensive Care Med 24:147-151
17. DeJonge E, Levi M, Berends F et al (1998) Impaired haemostasis by intravenous administration of a gelatin-based plasma expander in human subjects. Thromb Haemost 79:286-290
18. Strauss RG (1981) Review of the effects of hydroxyethyl starch on the blood coagulation system. Transfusion 21:299-309
19. Treib J, Haass A, Pindur G et al (1996) All medium starches are not the same: influence of hydroxyethyl substitution of hydroxyethhyl starch on plasma volume, hemorrheologic conditions, and coagulation. Transfusion 36:450-455

20. Treib J, Haass A, Pindur G (1997) Coagulation disorders caused by hydroxyethyl starch. Thromb Haemost 78:974-983
21. Boldt J, Zickmann B, Benson M et al (1992) Influence of 5 different priming on platelet function in patients undergoing cardiac surgery. Anesth Analg 74:219-225
22. Warren BB, Durieux ME (1996) Hydroxyethylstarch: safe or not? Anesth Analg 84:206-212
23. Schmand J, Ayala A, Chaudry IH (1994) Effects of trauma, duration of hypotension, and resuscitation regimen on cellular immunity after hemorrhagic shock. Crit Care Med 22:1076-1083
24. Dorman T, Breslow MJ (1994) Altered immune function after trauma and hemorrhage: what does it all mean? Crit Care Med 22:1069-1070
25. Chaudry IH, Ayala A (1993) Immune consequences of hypovolemic shock and resuscitation. Curr Opin Anaesth 6:385-392
26. Mariscalco MM (1993) Leukocytes and the inflammatory response. Crit Care Med 21:S347-S348
27. Williams TJ, Hellewell PG (1992) Endothelial cell biology. Am Rev Resp Dis 146:S45-S50
28. Springer TA (1990) Adhesion receptors of the immune system. Nature 346:425-434
29. Rothlein R, Mainolfi EA, Czajkowski M et al (1991) A form of circulating ICAM-1 in human serum. J Immunol 147:3788-3793
30. Seth R, Raymond FD, Makgoba MW (1991) Circulating ICAM-1 isoforms: diagnostic prospects for inflammatory and immune disorders. Lancet 338:83-84
31. Jochum M, Inthorn D, Waydhas Ch et al (1994) Diagnostic relevance of PMN elastase and soluble adhesion molecules in acute inflammation. Intensive Care Med 20:S102
32. Boldt J, Müller M, Heesen M et al (1996) Influence of different volume therapies and pentoxifylline infusion on circulating soluble adhesion molecules in critically ill patients. Crit Care Med 24:385-391

Chapter 8

Hydroxyethyl starch and coagulation

J. Treib, M.T. Grauer

Hydroxyethyl starch (HES) is one of the most frequently used volume replacement agents. Its advantages, such as high efficacy, few allergic reactions, low cost and general availability, are generally acknowledged. The main disadvantage of HES is its adverse effects on coagulation and resulting hemorrhagic complications. During recent years, studies have been carried out that attempted to examine how HES affects rheology and coagulation, to what extent these effects are clinically relevant and how they can be avoided. Since the first reports of bleeding complications were published in the 1980s, several new types of HES have entered the market, giving the physician a greater choice and the opportunity to avoid some of the undesired side effects of HES.

Here, we first give an overview of the pharmacology of the different types of HES. This is important for an understanding of the effects on coagulation, since the various types of HES can differ greatly in their pharmacokinetics, and it is the nature of the HES molecules that determine their clinical effect. In addition, we attempt to outline what is known about the effects of HES on coagulation and rheology. The conclusion seeks to give the clinician a few guidelines about which type of HES is preferable in clinical situations.

Clinical uses for hydroxyethyl starch

Hydroxyethyl starch is often used as a plasma substitute for therapy of hypovolemia after trauma, burns, infections or during surgery [1, 2]. It is also widely used for hemodilution treatment of cerebral ischemia and of retinal [3], otogenic [4] or peripheral [5] perfusion disturbances. In treatment of cerebral ischemia, a hypervolemic therapy protocol [6-8] has been shown to be more effective than an isovolemic infusion [9, 10]. Another indication is the hyperdynamic treatment of vasospasm in subarachnoid hemorrhage [11]. Some of these indications require relatively high dosages to ensure efficacy of therapy. However, during continuous treatment with large volumes of HES, disturbances of coagulation and hemorrhagic complications are not uncommon [12-15]. Trumble et al. [16] reported bleeding complications during hetastarch therapy of vasospasm in subarachnoid hemorrhage patients and recommended the use of plasma protein fraction instead. Van den Brink [17] observed coagulopathy under therapy with highly substituted medium molecular weight HES. These disturbances of the coagulation system were found to be due to an acquired von Willebrand syndrome [18-20]. This will be discussed below in greater detail.

Physical and chemical characteristics of hydroxyethyl starch

In order to understand the clinical differences between the different types of HES, it is important to take a closer look at the chemistry.

HES is a modified polymer of amylopectin, composed of glucose subunits, which are linked within the chain by α-1,4 glycoside bonds and at the branching points by α-1,6 bonds. The modification consists of adding hydroxyethyl groups to the glucose groups. Worldwide, many different HES preparations are used which differ mainly in four characteristics: concentration of HES in the solution, medium in vitro molecular weight (MW), degree of hydroxyethylation and pattern of hydroxyethylation.

Frequently used concentrations are 10%, 6% and 3%. The medium MW as indicated by the manufacturer gives an estimate of the average size of the molecules in daltons. HES molecules are not all the same size and the molecules in a preparation of HES show great polydispersity with respect not only to MW but also with respect to the pattern of hydroxyethylation. Molecule sizes follow a bell-shaped distribution and range from a few thousand daltons to a few million daltons. HES is divided into high MW (HMW), medium MW (MMW) and low MW (LMW) starch. The MW, are approximately 480 kDa, 200 KDa and 70 kDa, respectively. The MW is important because it is the number, and not the size, of the molecules that is responsible for the osmotic effect. At equal concentrations, the starch with a lower MW contains more osmotically active molecules.

Another important and somewhat complicated characteristic of HES is the degree and pattern of hydroxyethylation. To classify the product, one can measure how many hydroxyethyl groups are attached to the glucose subunits. The result, the degree of substitution, is a number between zero and one, typically ranging in HES between 0.4 and 0.7.

Besides determining how many glucose molecules are substituted, one can measure where they are substituted. The glucose groups can be hydroxyethylated at carbon 2, 3 or 6, depending on manufacturing. Because substitution occurs most frequently at position C2 and C6, HES is classified in general by the C2/C6 ratio, which indicates how many hydroxyethyl groups are attached at the C2 of glucose compared to C6. The C2/C6 ratio ranges from 4 to 13.

Both degree of substitution and C2/C6 ratio are clinically important. Starch without hydroxyethyl groups is rapidly degraded in the blood by amylases, and its half-life is short. Through hydroxyethylation, the breakdown of starch is inhibited considerably. This is probably due to steric hindrance of the enzymes through the hydroxyethylgroups. The more hydroxyethyl groups exist, and the higher the share of hydroxyethyl groups attached at C2, the longer the half-life of a starch [21]. In other words, the higher the degree of substitution and the higher the C2/C6 ratio, the slower starch is metabolized.

Pharmacokinetics of hydroxyethyl starch

As mentioned before, both degree of substitution and C2/C6 ratio are important for the pharmacokinetics of HES as well as for clinical practice. Immediately after the beginning of an infusion, the HES molecules are cleaved by α-amylases. This process generates new and smaller molecules, and the in vivo MW of HES begins to differ from the initial MW. However, for the clinical effects as well as the side effects of HES, such as the volume effect, and the effect on coagulation and rheology, it is the in vivo MW which is of decisive importance, not the initial in vitro MW. The in vivo MW depends partially on the initial size of the molecules, but also on the degree of substitution and the C2/C6 ratio.

Mishler and Ferber showed that, immediately after HES infusion, the MW distribution of the circulating molecules was much narrower and their average value was smaller than that of the infused solution [22, 23]. This indicates that small molecules with a MW less than about 50 000 daltons are cleared by renal excretion, and that larger molecules of HMW HES are hydrolyzed by amylases to generate new smaller molecules. The urinary excretion rate, for example, of the various HES solutions depends more on degree of substitution than on their in vitro MW [24].

The role of intravascular cleavage of HES is debated by some authors. For a MMW HES (HES 200/0.62) Baron et al. have demonstrated that intravascular hydrolysis was minimal [25]. In this theory, the reticulo-endothelial system (RES) plays a major role in the elimination of HES molecules with a high degree of substitution or a high C2/C6 ratio.

Effects of hydroxyethyl starch on coagulation

Bleeding complications after infusion of HMW HES (HES 480/0.7) have been reported repeatedly in the past. In a series of studies, the effects of five different HES preparations were examined [21, 26-31] The preparations included MMW HES, such as 10% HES 200/0.62 and 6% HES 200/0.62, two MMW starches with a lower degree of substitution of 0.5 and differing C2/C6 ratio (10% HES 200/0.5/6, 10% HES 200/0.5/13), and one LMW HES, 6% HES 70/0.5. During a 10-day hemodilution therapy in patients with cerebrovascular disorders, a total dose of approximately 7 500 ml of HES was infused. Parameters investigated included thromboplastin time (Quick), thrombin time and activated partial thromboplastin time (PTT) and factor VIII/von Willebrand factor (FVIII/vWF). Because the main reason for hemorrhagic complications under therapy with HES is the reduction in F VIII/vWF, the different FVIII/vWF subunits were also measured: factor VIII:C, von Willebrand Ristocetin cofactor and von Willebrand factor antigen. In general, the studies showed that the effects of HES on coagulation depend on the particular pharmacokinetics of each starch. Starches that are more difficult to degrade, for example starches with a high degree of substitution or a high C2/C6 ratio, lead to an accumulation of macromolecules, which in turn affect coagulation.

Thromboplastin time (Quick) is affected most by 10% HES 200/0.62. After a 10-day hemodilution therapy, the reduction reached approximately 20%. The other

MMW or LMW starch studies did not result in a clinically significant reduction of the thromboplastin time. These results are in agreement with earlier studies of the change in thromboplastin time after a 1-day HES therapy [32-35]. Thrombin time is affected in a similar manner. HES with a higher degree of substitution or a higher C2/C6 ratio (10% HES 200/0.62 and 10% HES 200/0.5/13) leads to a larger shortening of thrombin time and also to decrease in fibrinogen concentration. This is probably caused by an accelerated polymerization of fibrin and is of secondary relevance for hemostasis [33]. HES with a lower molecular weight or a lower degree of substitution or a lower C2/C6 ratio (10% HES 200/0.5/6 and 6% HES 70/0.5) does not affect fibrinogen concentration or thrombin time significantly.

Clinically more relevant are the changes in activated partial thromboplastin time (aPTT). After adminstration of HES that is difficult to degrade, such as HES 200/0.62 or HES 200/0.5/13, aPTT increased up to 40%. This increase points to an impairment of the intrinsic clotting system. It is caused mainly by a decrease in the concentration of FVIII/vWF, which is involved in the adhesion of platelets to injured blood vessels. Normally, a decrease in FVIII/vWF does not result in spontaneous hemorrhages, but can contribute to after bleedings, even from smaller injuries. Again, HES with a smaller molecular weight or HES that is easier to degrade (10% HES 200/0.5/6 and 6% HES 70/0.5) does not change aPTT beyond the dilution effect.

A more detailed vWF multimeric analysis showed that HES which is less degradable causes all multimers to decrease by approximately the same amount. The clotting disorder resulting from certain HES is therefore a quantitative effect, corresponding to a type I von Willebrand syndrome [28, 36, 37]. The precise pathomechanism of FVIII/vWF inhibition is unknown. In vitro studies are difficult to carry out and cannot entirely reproduce the in vivo mechanisms [38]. It is hypothesized that large HES molecules attach to FVIII/vWF, leading to an accelerated elimination of the complex. This hypothesis is supported by the fact that

Table 1. Influence of hydroxyethyl starch (HES) on coagulation during a 10-day hemodilution therapy

Type of HES	In vitro MW (kDa)	Degree of substitution	C2/C6 ratio	PTT	FVIII	vWF:AG
Rapidly degradable LMW HES	70	0.5	4	+4.0%	+8.2%	−1.9%
Rapidly degradable MMW HES	200	0.5	6	+7.9%	−7.9%	−6.1%
Slowly degradable MMW HES	200	0.5	13	+16.6%	−24.6%	−17.6%
Slowly degradable MMW HES	200	0.62	10	+42.8%	−70.4%	−83.6%

FVIII, factor VIII; *vWF:AG,* von Willebrand factor antigen

Siostrzonek et al. [39] were able to show a factor VIII-IgG paraprotein complex which leads to an accelerated elimination of FVIII/vWF and to an acquired von Willebrand syndrome. Both types of acquired von Willebrand syndrome can be treated with desmopressin (DDAVP), which causes a release of factor VIII from the endothelium [20].

Because the very large HES molecules lead to a decrease in FVIII/vWF, hemorrhagic problems are correlated with a larger dose of HES, greater numbers of large molecules, a higher degree of substitution and a higher C2/C6 ratio of the starch. These problems can be avoided by using an appropriate starch with a low in vivo molecular weight (Table 1).

Hydroxyethyl starch and rheology

Similar to coagulation, the rheological parameters hematocrit, plasma viscosity and erythrocyte aggregation are affected differently by the different types of HES. For the macrocirculation, hematocrit and the viscosity of full blood are of decisive importance. For the microcirculation, hematocrit is not as important as erythrocyte aggregation and plasma viscosity.

The effect on hematocrit depends on the volume effect, which in turn depends on the concentration of HES and the number of oncotically active molecules; 10% HES 200/0.5 solutions have an additional volume binding effect of 50%-100% of the infused volume [40]. For this reason, 10% HES solutions are usually administered together with electrolyte solution. In our studies, 10% HES 200/0.62 had the most pronounced and longest lasting volume effect. However, the volume effect of the LMW HES was relatively large, considering that only a 6% solution was used. LMW HES contains smaller, but more, molecules resulting in a satisfactory volume effect despite the lower concentration, but the duration of the volume effect is shorter.

Erythrocyte aggregation is aided by a reversible bridge-binding of the erythrocytes, which can approach each other only up to 30 nm because of repulsing Coulomb forces. Erythrocytes aggregate if larger molecules, such as fibrinogen or HES, bridge the distance between the erythrocyte membranes [8]. By contrast, smaller molecules can push away the larger, aggregation-supporting molecules and therefore lower erythrocyte aggregation. For this reason, high doses of HES with a larger in vivo molecular weight (such as HES 200/0.62 or 480/0.7) increase erythrocyte aggregation, whereas low in vivo molecular weight HES (200/0.5 or 70/0.5) lowers the tendency of erythrocytes to aggregate.

Plasma viscosity is another parameter which is important for the microcirculation. Following the Fahraeus-Lindqvist effect, the effective viscosity of blood in the capillaries approaches the viscosity of plasma. The latter depends to a large extent on macromolecules in the plasma, such as fibrinogen, but is also affected by starch molecules. The accumulation of larger HES molecules (MW larger than 100 kDa) in the plasma, which occurs during administration of HMW HES or slowly degradable medium molecular weight HES increases plasma viscosity [26, 27]. HES with an in vivo molecular weight less than 90 kDa (i. e. HES 200/0.5 or 70/0.5) lowers

Table 2. Influence of hydroxyethyl starch (HES) on hemorheology during a 10-day hemodilution therapy

Type of HES	In vitro MW (kDa)	Degree of substitution	C2/C6 ratio	In vivo MW [kD]	Plasma viscosity	P value
Rapidly degradable LMW HES	70	0.5	4	57.5	-1.5%	n.s.
Rapidly degradable MMW HES	200	0.5	6	84.1	+3.1%	n.s.
Slowly degradable MMW HES	200	0.5	13	95.0	+10.1%	<0.01
Slowly degradable MMW HES	200	0.62	10	120.6	+18.5%	<0.01

plasma viscosity [27]. Table 2 summarizes the most important findings. Overall, medium molecular weight HES and HES that is more easily degradable have more favourable effects on rheological parameters. HMW HES increases plasma viscosity and erythrocyte aggregation.

Conclusions

Each HES preparation is polydisperse and contains a range of molecules from a few thousand to a few million dalton. The HES molecules with high molecular weights cause the main undesired effects of HES, namely the impairment of coagulation, unfavourable influences on rheology and accumulation of macromolecules. HES molecules with high or medium molecular weight accumulate, if the starch is difficult to metabolize. This is the case for starches with a high degree of substitution or a high C2/C6 ratio or a combination of these parameters. To enable easy elimination, the larger molecules have to cleaved by α-amylases, until their size is smaller than the renal threshold.

A one-time administration of any starch is generally safe as far as coagulation problems are concerned. When administered over a longer period of time or in greater volumes, starches that are difficult to degrade can cause hemorrhagic problems through a reduction of FVIII/vWF leading in some instances to an acquired von Willebrand syndrome type I. Hemorrhagic complications and negative rheologic effects under therapy with HES can be avoided by selecting starches with a low in vivo molecular weight.

In summary, HESs that have a lower initial molecular weight and a degree and pattern of hydroxyethylation that allows easier degradation, such as HES 200/0.5/6 or HES 70/0.5, lead to fewer undesired effects.

References

1. London MJ, Ho Js, Triedman JK, Verrier ED, Levine J, Merrick SH, Hanley FL, Browner WS, Mangono DT (1989) A randomized clinical trial of 10% pentastarch (low molecular weight hydroxyethyl starch) versus 5% albumin for plasma volume expansion after cardiac operations. J Thorac Cardiovasc Surg 97:785-797
2. Shoemaker WC, Kram HB (1990) Effects of crystalloids and colloids on hemodynamics, oxygen transport and outcome in high-risk surgical patients. In: Simmons RC, Udekuo AS (eds) Debates in clinical surgery. Yearbook, Chicago, pp 263-316
3. Arend O, Hoberg A, Bertram B, Reim M, Wolf S (1991) Hemodilution in acute arterial circulatory disorders of the retina. Acta-Med-Austriaca 18(Suppl 1):66-68
4. Zennaro O, Dauman R, Poisot A, Esteben D, Duclose JY, Bertrand B, Cros AM, Milacic M, Bebear JP (1993) Value of the association of normovolemic dilution and hyperbaric oxygenation in the treatment of sudden deafness. A retrospective study. Ann Otolaryngol Chir Cervicofac 110:162-169
5. Kiesewetter H, Jung F, Blume J, Gerhards M (1987) Hämodilution bei Patienten mit peripherer arterieller Verschlußkrankheit im Stadium IIb: prospektiver randomisierter Doppelblind-Vergleich von mittelmolekularer Hydroxyethylstärke und kleinmolekularer Dextranlösung. Klin Wschr 65:324-330
6. The Hemodilution in Stroke Study Group (1989) Hypervolemic hemodilution treatment of acute stroke. Results of a randomized multicenter trial using pentastarch. Stroke 20:317-323
7. Koller M, Haenny P, Hess K, Weniger D, Zangger P (1990) Adjusted hypervolemic hemodilution in acute ischemic stroke. Stroke 21:1429-1434
8. Haass A, Stoll M, Treib J (1992) Hemodilution in cerebral circulatory disturbances: indications, implementation additional drug treatment and alternatives. In Hemodilution. New aspects in the management of circulatory blood flow. Improvement of macro- and microcirculation. Springer-Verlag, Berlin Heidelberg New York, pp 53-114
9. Scandinavian Stroke Study Group (1987) Multicenter trial of hemodilution in acute ischemic stroke. Stroke 18:691-699
10. Italian Acute Stroke Study Group (1988) Hemodilution in acute stroke. Results of the Italian hemodilution trial. The Lancet 13:318-320
11. Mori K, Arai H, Nakajima K, Tajima A, Maeda M (1995) Hemorheological and hemodynamic analysis of hypervolemic hemodilution therapy for cerebral vasospasm after aneurysmal subarachnoid hemorrhage. Stroke 26:1620-1626
12. Symington BE (1986) Hetastarch and bleeding complication. Ann Intern Med 105:627-628
13. Cully MD, Larson CP, Silverberg GD (1987) Hetastarch coagulopathy in a neurosurgical patient. Anaesthesiology 66:707-708
14. Damon L, Adams M, Stricker RB, Ries C (1987) Intracranial bleeding during treatment with hydroxyethyl starch. N Engl J Med 317:964-965
15. Chang JC, Gross HM, Jang NS (1990) Disseminated intravascular coagulation due to intravenous administration of hetastarch. Am J Sci 300:301-303
16. Trumble ER, Muizelaar JP, Myseros JS, Choi SC, Warren BB (1995) Coagulopathy with the use of hetastarch in the treatment of vasospasm. J Neurosurg 82:44-47
17. van den Brink WA, van Genderen P, Thijsse WJ, Michiels JJ (1996) Hetastarch coagulopathy. J Neurosurg 85:367
18. Sanfelippo MJ, Suberviola PD, Geimer NF (1987) Development of a von Willebrand like syndrome after prolonged use of hydroxyethyl starch. Am J Clin Pathol 88:653-655

19. Dalrymple HM, Aitchison R, Collins P, Sekhar M, Colvin B (1992) Hydroxyethyl starch induced acquired von Willebrand's disease. Clin Lab Haematol 14:209-211

20. Conroy JM, Fishman RL, Reeves ST, Pinosky ML, Lazzarchick J (1996) The effect of desmopressin and 6% hydroxyethyl starch on factor VIII:C. Anaesth Analg 83:804-807

21. Treib J, Haass A, Pindur G, Seyfert UT, Treib W, Grauer MT, Jung F, Wenzel E, Schimrigk K (1995) HES 200/0.5 is not HES 200/0.5. Influence of the C2/C6 hydroxyethylation ratio of hydroxyethyl starch (HES) on hemorheology, coagulation and elimination kinetics. Thromb Haemost 74:1452-1456

22. Mishler JM, Ricketts CR, Parkhouse EJ (1980) Post-transfusion survival of hydroxyethyl starch 450/0.70 in man: a long-term study. J Clin Pathol 33:155-159

23. Ferber HP, Nitsch E, Forster H (1985) Studies on hydroxyethyl starch. Part II: Changes of the molecular weight distribution for hydroxyethyl starch types 450/0.7, 450/0.5, 450/0.3, 300/0.4, 200/0.7, 200/0.5, 200/0.3 and 200/0.1 after infusion in serum and urine of volunteers. Arzneimittelforschung 35:615-622

24. Korttila K, Grohn P, Gordin A, Sundberg S, Salo H, Nissinen E, Mattila MA (1984) Effect of hydroxyethyl starch and dextran on plasma volume and blood hemostasis and coagulation. J Clin Pharmacol 24:273-282

25. Degrémont AC, Ismail M, Arthaud M, Oulare B, Mundler O, Paris M, Baron JF (1995) Mechanisms of postoperative prolonged plasma volume expansion with low molecular weight hydroxyethyl starch (HES 200/0.62, 6%). Intensive Care Med 21:577-583

26. Treib J, Haass A, Pindur G, Grauer MT, Wenzel E, Schimrigk K (1996) All medium starches are not the same. Influence of degree of substitution of hydroxyethyl starch on plasma volume, hemorheologic conditions, and coagulation. Transfusion 36:450-455

27. Treib J, Haass A, Pindur G, Grauer MT, Seyfert UT, Treib W, Wenzel E, Schimrigk K (1996) Influence of low molecular weight hydroxyethyl starch on hemostasis and hemorheology. Haemostasis 26:258-265

28. Treib J, Haass A, Pindur G, Miyachita C, Grauer MT, Jung F, Wenzel E, Schimrigk K (1996) Highly substituted hydroxyethyl starch (HES 200/0.62) leads to a type I von Willebrand syndrome after repeated administration. Haemostasis 26:210-213

29. Treib J, Haass A, Pindur G, Grauer MT, Treib W, Wenzel E, Schimrigk K (1997) Increased hemorrhagic risk after repeated infusion of highly substituted medium molecular weight hydroxyethyl starch. Drug Res 47:18-22

30. Treib J, Haass A, Pindur G, Grauer MT, Wenzel E, Schimrigk K (1997) Avoiding an impairment of F VIII:C by using hydroxyethyl starch with a low in vivo molecular weight. Anesth Analg 84:1391

31. Treib J, Haass A, Pindur G (1997) Coagulation disorders caused by hydroxyethyl starch. Thromb Haemost 78:974-983

32. Peter K, Gander HP, Lutz H, Nold W, Strosiek U (1975) Die Beeinflussung der Blutgerinnung durch Hydroxyäthylstärke. Anaesthesist 24:219-224

33. Vinazzer H, Bergmann H (1975) Zur Beeinflussung postoperativer Änderungen der Blutgerinnung durch Hydroxyäthylstärke. Anaesthesist 24:517-520

34. Probst W (1988) Elohäst (Hydroxyethylstärke 6% 200/0.60-0.66) bei akuten ischämischen cerebralen Durchblutungsstörungen. Elohäst Workshop, pp 11-12

35. Reiger I (1988) Erfahrungen mit Elohäst (Hydroxyethylstärke 6% 200/0.60-0.66) in der Therapie des Cerebralinsults. Elohäst Workshop, p 10

36. Ruggeri ZM (1994) Pathogenesis and classification of von Willebrand disease. Haemostasis 24:265-275

37. Zimmerman TS, Ruggeri ZM (1983) Von Willebrand's Disease. Clin Haematol 12:175-200

38. Grauer MT, Treib J (1998) The effect of HES on coagulation is difficult to assess in vitro. Br J Anaesth 80:125-126
39. Siostrzonek P, Niessner H, Deutsch E, Lechner K, Korninger C, Pabinger I, Heinz R (1985) Vier Fälle mit erworbenem von Willebrand-Syndrom und monoklonaler Gammopathie. Langzeitverlauf sowie diagnostische und therapeutische Problematik. In: Landbeck G (ed) Hämophilie Symposium. Springer-Verlag, Berlin Heidelberg New York, pp 248-256
40. Kohler H, Zschiedrich H, Clasen R, Linfante A, Gamm H (1982) The effects of 500 ml 10% hydroxyethyl starch 200/0.5 and 10% dextran 40 on blood volume, colloid osmotic pressure and renal function in human volunteers. Anaesthesist 31:61-67

Chapter 9

Colloid-induced renal complications

J.F. BARON

Normovolemic hemodilution with colloids is recommended in a wide range of ischemic conditions, such as acute stroke, peripheral vascular disease and hearing loss, to improve microcirculatory perfusion and collateral flow. Since this particular category of patients usually has generalized atherosclerosis, often with some degree of pre-existing latent renal disease, it is not surprising that the colloids, albumin, dextran and hydroxyethyl starch (HES) are occasionally associated with the development of acute renal failure, particularly if dosage recommendations are not followed [1]. More recently, several publications have focused on another category of patients at risk, brain-dead donors for kidney transplantation [2].

Acute renal failure following infusion of colloids

Initially, this complication has only been described with dextrans. Within certain narrow, particularly high-risk subgroups, such as acute stroke, stage III and IV arteritis, the reported incidence of acute renal failure associated with dextran therapy ranged from virtually 0% in 500 patients on dextran 40, reported by Gottstein [3], to 4.3% in 207 patients, reported by Biesenbach [1]. The only evident, but possibly decisive, difference in these two reports concerns hydration: Gottstein's patients received an additional 250 ml 20% mannitol plus at least 7000 ml crystalloids or oral water daily to maintain adequate urine output.

A review of 23 published case reports published by Matheson [4] suggested that most of the cases of colloid-induced acute renal failure shared several risk factors: 1) they generaly involve elderly patients; 2) the patients received colloids for non-surgical reasons, i.e., claudication, stroke, sudden hearing loss; 3) the patients had preexisting or latent renal disease; 4) the patients were dehydrated with low urine output prior to colloid administration and had received high doses of 10% dextran 40 over several days.

Several hypotheses have been formulated to explain acute renal failure following dextran administration: direct toxicity, accumulation of low molecular weight fractions in the tubules and, more recently, hyperoncotic renal failure.

Low molecular weight dextran is a mixture of dextrose polymers with an average molecular weight of 40 000 (range: 10 000 to 80 000). In normal subjects, the components with the lowest molecular weight are excreted by the kidney within 12-24 h. The largest components may be retained in plasma or interstitial compartments for weeks. The chemical toxicity of dextran is low although it may induce vacuolization of proximal tubular cells [5]. These osmotic nephrosis-ike lesions have been reported with other colloids such as hydroxyethyl starches (HES) [6] and gelatins [7]. Initially, these lesions were considered as responsible for impairement of renal function. However, the lesions were also observed with agents that do not induce acute renal failure, such as mannitol and glucose [7].

Mailloux et al. suggested that direct toxicity was unlikely since in laboratory animals, dextran can induce acute renal failure within minutes after it is administered [8, 9]. In this setting, however, a prerequisite for the development of renal failure is severe constriction of the renal artery or severe hypovolemia as a consequence of noncompensated blood withdrawal. Mailloux et al. suggested that the combination of a decreased glomerular pressure with a maximal reabsorption of water may induce the accumulation in the tubule of the low molecular weight fraction of dextran with local hyperviscosity and precipitation.

Ten years later, a case report published by Moran et al. demonstrated the reversibility of acute renal failure by plasmapheresis [10]. This observation has been confirmed by several other publications [11-14], and has led to the formulation of another explanation for colloid-induced acute renal failure, the hyperoncotic mechanism. In the initial case report of Moran et al., it was demonstrated that a high plasma concentration of dextrans, inducing a high plasma colloido-osmotic pressure, counteracts the opposing hydraulic filtration pressure in the glomerulus. Indeed, the rate of glomerular filtration is governed by the imbalance between positive hydraulic forces that promote fluid movement into Bowman's space and negative oncotic forces that retard such movement [15, 16]. The glomerular filtration rate (GFR) may be expressed as $GFR = Kf (\Delta P - \Delta \Pi)$ where Kf is the glomerular ultrafiltration coefficient, ΔP is the mean difference in hydraulic pressure, and $\Delta \Pi$ is the mean difference in oncotic pressure. Because glomerular filtrate is essentially free of protein, the value for $\Delta \Pi$ is determined primarily by oncotic pressure within the glomerular capillary. Acute renal failure induced by ischemia or cellular toxins is characterized by alterations in glomerular hemodynamics. Net transglomerular hydraulic pressure may be reduced by either a rise in proximal tubular pressure or a fall in the hydraulic pressure in the glomerular capillary. Diminished glomerular permeability and tubuloglomerular feedback activation may also contribute to the reduction in the GFR [17]. Back-leak of filtrate across a damaged tubular epithelium can further reduce renal excretory capacity [18]. The equation shows that if the oncotic forces equal or exceed the hydraulic forces, glomerular filtration will cease. As protein-free glomerular filtrate is formed, the distal intracapillary oncotic pressure rises sufficiently to stop filtration [16]. Theoretically, an accumulation in plasma of any unfilterable, osmotically active substance could likewise induce cessation of glomerular filtration.

Because pressure within the glomerular capillary and proximal tubule cannot actually be measured in humans, accurate determination of the minimal transcapillary hydraulic pressure required to form glomerular filtrate is difficult. The patient of Moran et al. [10] provided a unique opportunity to make such an estimation. One might consider a hypothetical situation in which renal perfusion pressure is stable in the setting of anuria induced by elevated plasma oncotic pressure. If oncotic pressure is slowly reduced, urine flow will return when the net glomerular transcapillary hydraulic pressure just exceeds the oncotic pressure in the afferent arteriole of patent nephrons. The patient had no urine output when the total oncotic pressure was 28.7 mm Hg, and urine output returned when the oncotic pressure was 26.9 mm Hg. Therefore, a range of 27-29 mm Hg probably encompassed the minimal value of the transmembrane difference in hydraulic pressure necessary to form glomerular filtrate (Fig. 1).

This syndrome has been termed "hyperoncotic acute renal failure" [10]. The presence of anuria is not a diagnostic criterion. The patient's renal insufficiency developed over several days, initially during a period of nonoliguria. Presumably, the nephrons became nonfunctional progressively. Such a sequence may occur commonly, with its cause mistakenly attributed to other factors. One might speculate that other subjects, such as those with hyperproteinemia, could also be at risk for hyperoncotic renal dysfunction.

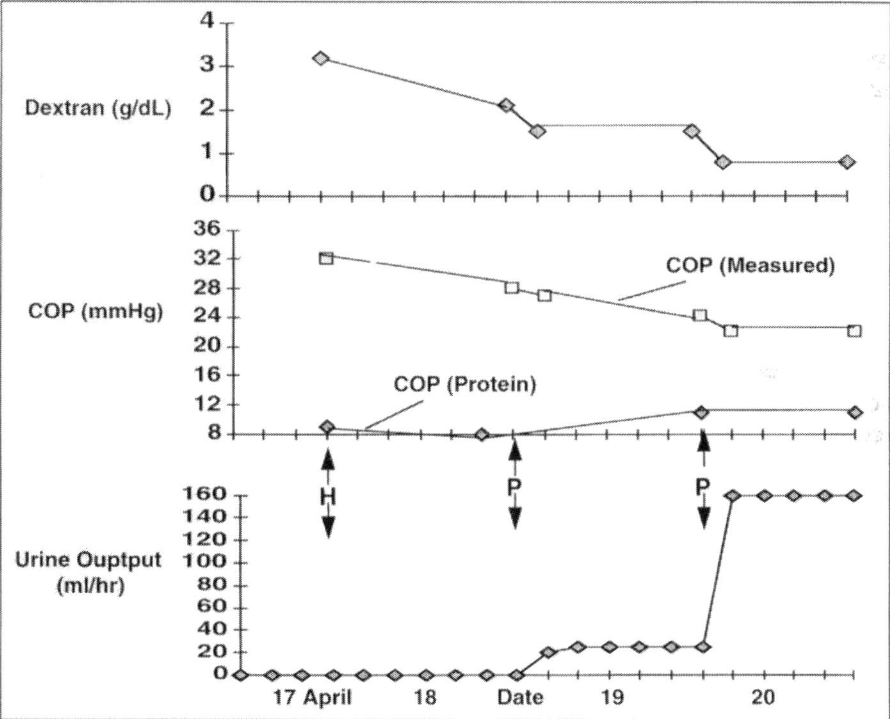

Fig. 1. Changes in dextran concentration, colloid osmotic pressure (COP) and urine output associated with hemodialysis and plasmapheresis (P). The last plasmapheresis demonstrates the mechanism of hyperoncotic acute renal failure. The patient had no urine output when the total oncotic pressure was 28.7 mm Hg, and urine output returned when the oncotic pressure was 26.9 mm Hg. Therefore, a range of 27-29 mm Hg probably encompassed the minimal value of the transmembrane difference in hydraulic pressure necessary to form glomerular filtrate. (Modified from [10])

This hypothesis has been reinforced by publication of additional cases following not only dextran but also HES [19], gelatin [20] and concentrated albumin [21] administration. Most of these cases have also confirmed the beneficial effect of plasmapheresis [11, 12, 14]. Until recently, it had been assumed that HES was relatively free of these problems in conjunction with its use in hemodilution. Within the last few years, however, the German health authorities began receiving several reports which also implicated HES in this context, as represented by Waldhausen et al. [19]. It is now known that all hyperoncotic colloid solutions, 20% albumin [21], 10% HES 200 [19] and 10% dextran 40, can induce acute renal failure. Acute renal failure has also been documented for 6% hetastarch [22] and 3.5% gelatin [20], but not for 6% dextran 70 or 3% dextran 60, nor for 5% albumin. It is likely that the risk of high plasma colloido-osmotic pressure is higher with colloids having either a high concentration (dextran 10%, HES 10%) or a high in vivo molecular weight responsible for plasma accumulation (hetastarch and elohes 6%).

In patients receiving colloids, particularly those with obstructive vascular disease, daily postoperative assessment of renal function is prudent. If renal function deteriorates and oligoanuria that is unresponsive to diuretic treatment occurs, direct measurement of colloid osmotic pressure is indicated. If the pressure is disproportionately elevated, the infusion of colloids should be stopped. If the decline in renal function is progressive, plasmapheresis may be the appropriate therapy.

Adverse effects of colloids on transplanted organs

In 1993, Legendre et al. reported osmotic nephrosis-like lesions in most of the transplanted kidneys subsequently biopsied at Necker Hospital in Paris [6]. In an historical study, they founded that 80% of the kidneys transplanted at their center during 1992, when HES was routinely administered to brain-dead donors, had osmotic nephrosis-like lesions in biopsies taken 6 weeks after transplantation. Only 14% of the kidneys transplanted during 1990, prior to implementation of HES administration, revealed such lesions upon biopsy. Demographic data, the use of contrast media and choice of preservation solution were similar in the two groups. The incidence of osmotic nephrosis-like lesions was not influenced by cold ischemia time, presence and length of delayed graft function, or immunosuppressive regimen, especially, the use of cyclosporine. Conversely, these lesions had no significant deleterious influence on the occurrence of delayed graft function and serum creatinine at 3 and 6 months post-transplantation. However, osmotic nephrosis-like lesions might be long-lasting since in three patients they were still present at 3 months post-transplantation on routine renal biopsy. In the patients without osmoticy nephrosis-like lesions no kidney was lost, whereas among those with such lesions, seven of 31 were lost. Legendre et al. went on to recommend the avoidance of HES in potential organ donors.

Although accepting that the adverse effect on renal transplant survival is a new finding, the German drug committee did not feel that there is yet sufficient evidence to issue an official drug alert. They claim that Legendre's publication, upon which the warning was based, is a retrospective case repot analysis without statistical evaluation and therefore has no scientific value.

Thus, a prospective randomized study was initiated by Cittanova et al. [2]. The main objective of the study was to determine the effects on renal function in kidney transplant recipients of administering HES or gelatin to brain dead donors. Over 18 months, 121 brain-dead donors were admitted in their hospital. Patients who recieved iodinated contast media were excluded. Multiple organ harvesting was possible in only 29 patients including 27 kidney donors, 15 in the HES group and 12 in the gelatin group, leading to, respectively, 27 and 20 kidney recipients in the HES group and gelatin group. In the HES group, brain-dead patients needing colloids received HES up to the maximal dose of 33 ml/kg and then gelatin. In the gelatin group, brain-dead donors received only gelatin for plasma volume expansion. There were no significant differences in age, cause and duration of brain-death, need for dopamine or other cardiovascular support, transfusion requirement and preoperative serum creatinine between the two groups. One out of 20 (5%) kidney recipients in the gelatin group needed extrarenal hemodialysis or hemofiltration within the first week after transplantation compared with nine out of 27 (33%) in the HES group ($p<0.03$). Serum creatinine for the first 10 days after transplantation was significantly lower in the gelatin group than in the HES group (Fig. 2). Nine real biopsy specimens were examined, six in the gelatin group. All three specimens

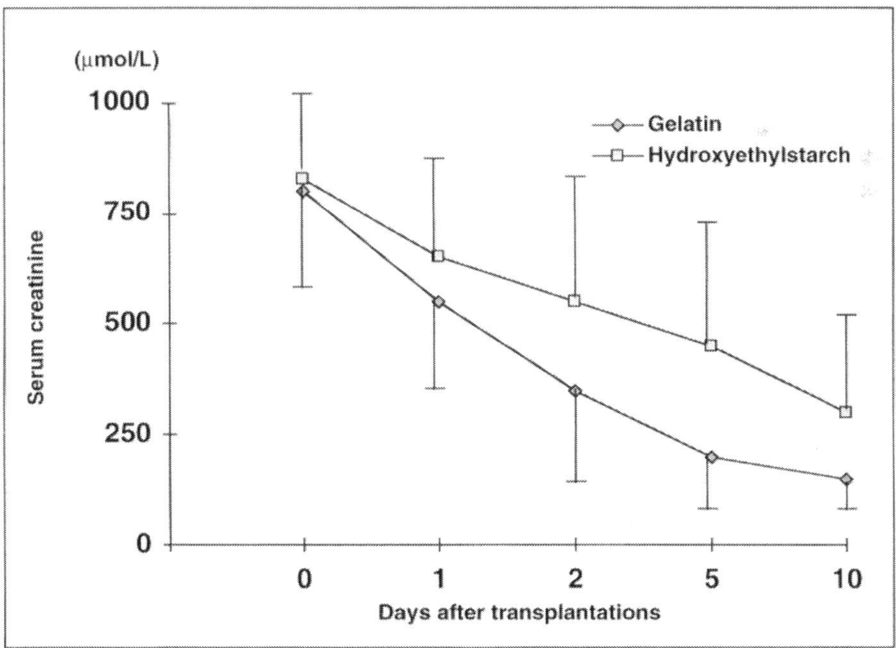

Fig. 2. Serum creatinine after kidney transplantation (mean, SD). (Modified from [2])

in the HES group had osmotic nephrosis-like lesions. This prospective randomized study seems to confirm the results of the earlier study of Legendre et al.

However, Coronel et al reported controversial data [23]. They analyzed 24 renal transplant biopsy specimens taken 15 min after kidney reperfusion. They classified these into two groups according to the use of HES or not for resuscitation of the brain-dead donors. Four out of 16 (25%) patients who received HES had osmotic nephrosis-like lesions and two out of eight (25%) patients who had not received HES had the same lesions. In addition, the authors did not observe any functional impact of HES administration on postoperative kidney graft function. In this study, the osmotic nephrosis-like lesions were less frequent (25%) than reported by Legendre and Cittanova [2, 6]. For Coronel, there is no specific reason to attribute the lesions to HES. Indeed, none of these three studies have identified HES in the vacuoles seen on kidney biopsies, indicating that a direct relationship with HES has still to be established. Coronel et al concluded that the hemodynamic status of the donor is still central to the occurrence of these lesions [23]. It could also be suggested that high colloido-osmotic pressure following colloids administration is an important mechanism which may in part explain acute renal failure after kidney transplantation. Plasma colloido-osmotic pressure may be of critical value when renal perfusion pressure is compromised after ischemic reperfusion lesions, and this information is never available in these studies.

In addition, all these studies are limited to very small number patients and a large scale-study is still needed to make definite conclusions. Until that point, it can be cautiously recommended not to use HES or dextrans as plasma volume expanders in brain-dead donors and in kidney transplant recipients.

Conclusions

Most of the cases of colloid-induced acute renal failure share several risk factors. They generaly involve elderly patients. The patients have received colloids for non-surgical reasons, such as claudication, stroke, sudden hearing loss. The patients have preexisting or latent renal disease. The patients have been dehydrated with low urine output prior to colloid administration and have received high doses of colloids over several days. It has now been demonstrated that a high plasma concentration of colloids, inducing a high plasma colloido-osmotic pressure, counteracts the opposing hydraulic filtration pressure in the glomerulus. This syndrome is termed hyperoncotic acute renal failure.

Initially, hyperoncotic acute renal failure has been only described with dextrans. It is now known that all hyperoncotic colloid solutions, 20% albumin, 10% HES 200 and 10% dextran 40, can induce acute renal failure. Acute renal failure has also been documented for 6% hetastarch and gelatin, but not for 6% dextran 70 or 3% dextran 60, nor for 5% albumin. It is likely that the risk of high plasma colloido-osmotic pressure is greater with colloids having either a high concentration (dextran 10%, HES 200 10%, albumin 20%) or a high in vivo molecular weight responsible for plasma accumulation (hetastarch or elohes 6%).

In patients receiving colloids, particularly those with obstructive vascular dis-

Table 1. Incidence of osmotic nephrosis-like lesions in patients with transplanted kidneys exposed to HES or not exposed to HES is not significantly different. (From [23])

	Osmotic nephrosis –	Osmotic nephrosis +
HES –	6	2 (25%)
HES +	12	4 (25%)

HES, hydroxyethyl starch

ease, daily postoperative assessment of renal function is prudent. If renal function deteriorates and oligoanuria that is unresponsive to diuretic treatment occurs, direct measurement of colloid osmotic pressure is indicated. If the pressure is disproportionately elevated, the infusion of colloids should be stopped. If the decline in renal function is progressive, plasmapheresis may be the appropriate therapy (Tab. 1)

References

1. Biesenbach G, Kaiser W, Zazgornik J (1997) Incidence of acute oligoanuric renal failure in dextran 40 treated patients with acute ischemic stroke stage III or IV. Ren Fail 19:69-75
2. Cittanova ML, Leblanc I, Legendre C, Mouquet C, Riou B, Coriat P (1996) Effect of hydroxyethylstarch in brain-dead kidney donors on renal function in kidney-transplant recipients. Lancet 348:1620-1622
3. Gottstein U (1974) Treatment of inadequate cerebral circulation. A critical review. Internist 15:575-587
4. Matheson NA, Diomi P (1970) Renal failure after the administration of dextran 40. Surg Gynecol Obstet 131:661-668
5. Diomi P, Ericsson JL, Matheson NA (1970) Effects of dextran 40 on urine flow and composition during renal hypoperfusion in dogs with osmotic nephrosis. Ann Surg 172:813-824
6. Legendre C, Thervet E, Page B, Percheron A, Noel LH, Kreis H (1993) Hydroxyethyl-starch and osmotic-nephrosis-like lesions in kidney transplantation (Letter). Lancet 342:248-249
7. Kief H (1969) Morphological findings following single or multiple administration of gelatin plasma substitutes. Bibl Haematol 33:367-379
8. Mailloux L, Swartz CD, Capizzi R, Kim KE, Onesti G, Ramirez O, Brest AN (1967) Acute renal failure after administration of low-molecular weight dextran. N Engl J Med 277:1113-1118
9. Chinitz JL, Kim KE, Onesti G, Swartz C (1971) Pathophysiology and prevention of dextran-40-induced anuria. J Lab Clin Med 77:76-87
10. Moran M, Kapsner C (1987) Acute renal failure associated with elevated plasma oncotic pressure. N Engl J Med 317:150-153
11. Ferraboli R, Malheiro PS, Abdulkader RC, Yu L, Sabbaga E, Burdmann EA (1997) Anuric acute renal failure caused by dextran 40 administration. Ren Fail 19:303-306
12. Kurnik BR, Singer F, Groh WC (1991) Case report: dextran-induced acute anuric renal failure. Am J Med Sci 302:28-30

13. Zwaveling JH, Meulenbelt J, van Xanten NH, Hene RJ (1989) Renal failure associated with the use of dextran-40. Neth J Med 35:321-326
14. Van Den Berg CJ, Pineda AA (1980) Plasma exchange in the treatment of acute renal failure due to low molecular-weight dextran. Mayo Clin Proc 55:387-389
15. Myers BD (1983) Pathogenesis of acute renal failure in man. Kidney 16:37-41
16. Deen WM, Robertson CR, Brenner BM (1972) A model of glomerular ultrafiltration in the rat. Am J Physiol 223:1178-1183
17. Stein JH (1977) The glomerulus in acute renal failure. J Lab Clin Med 90:227-230
18. Blantz RC, Pelayo JC (1984) A functional role for the tubuloglomerular feedback mechanism. Kidney Int 25:739-746
19. Waldhausen P, Kiesewetter H, Leipnitz G, Scielny J, Jung F, Bambauer R, von Blohn G (1991) Hydroxyethyl starch-induced transient renal failure in preexisting glomerular damage. Acta Med Austriaca 1:52-55
20. Hussain SF, Drew PJ (1989) Acute renal failure after infusion of gelatins. BMJ 299:1137-1138
21. Rozich JD, Paul RV (1989) Acute renal failure precipitated by elevated colloid osmotic pressure. Am J Med 87:359-360
22. Haskell LP, Tannenberg AM (1988) Elevated urinary specific gravity in acute oliguric renal failure due to hetastarch administration. State J Med 88:387-388
23. Coronel B, Mercatello A, Martin X, Lefrancois N (1997) Hydroxyethylstarch and renal function in kidney transplant recipients (Letter). Lancet 349:884

Chapter 10

Airway management

F. Agrò

The development of intubation techniques has been very important to the history of anesthesiology and critical care. Over the past decade significant advances have been achieved in the field of airway management. For example, greater attention has been paid to proper evaluation of the risks of difficult or impossible ventilation and/or intubation, as well as to the marketing of new devices that aid in unpredicted difficult intubations (laryngeal mask airway, Combitube, LMA-Fastrach, etc.). In addition, the kinds and the quality available of the facilities for assisting patients with airway problems have been improved. Tracheal intubation is necessary in numerous circumstances: respiratory or circulatory failure, neurological accidents, airway protection of patients at risk of bronchial inhalation, general anesthesia in paralyzed patients, etc. But this simple maneuver may sometimes be extremely difficult or even impossible, accounting for the numerous deaths and pathologies due to prolonged hypoxia. Unfortunately, a significant number of problems during airway emergency is iatrogenic: every year about 600 [1] patients die due to failed airway management in emergencies all over the world. The incidence of difficult intubations is 2.3% of all patients [2], and up to 10% of patients suffering from otolaryngologic pathologies [3]. Intubation failures range from 0.04% of all patients to 0.35% of obstetric patients [4].

As in outpatient medicine the available means are limited, there is a higher incidence of difficult intubation. In addition, some kinds of lesions can make tracheal intubation difficult in polytraumatized patients, especially as far as maxillofacial and cervical rachis traumas are concerned. After a severe maxillofacial trauma, intubation may be difficult because of massive bleeding or anatomical impairment. In order to evaluate existing difficulties, an anesthesiological clinical test is absolutely necessary. In the case of unpredicted difficulties, based on the clinical test or in an emergency, it is essential that clinicians have a perfectly codified – and not improvised – procedure.

Difficult airway

Some 33% of anesthesiological accidents involving cerebral impairment or even death are due to failed airway management [5]. An incidence ranging from 1% to 3.5% is reported in the literature [6], but is probably underestimated. This figure rises up to 1/300 in obstetric patients (Lyons G, personal communication) as they have increased water retention and therefore tissue edema.

Definition

A difficult airway, according to the American Society of Anesthesiology (ASA), is when an experienced anesthesiologist finds it difficult to perform a mask ventilation, a tracheal intubation, or both; a difficult mask ventilation occurs when a trained anesthesiologist is unable to maintain 90% SpO_2 using 100% O_2 with a facemask; a difficult intubation is one which occurs after two (according to the French school) or three (according to the UK school) attempts, or when it takes more than 10 min and is not the same as a difficult laryngoscopy, which corresponds to Cormack and Lehane Grade 3 or 4 [7].

Failed intubation, meant as giving up further attempts, has a high incidence (1:2 000) and is however higher today than in the past, since anesthesiologists are more cautious.

A failed tracheal intubation, with difficult ventilation, has an incidence of 1:10 000 [5].

Predicting a difficult intubation

To identify those patients at risk of difficult intubation is an essential part of the anesthesiological examination, for it can reduce both mortality and morbidity related to difficult airway. If the preoperative examination is correctly carried out, 98% of such cases will be predicted [8]. Even though this figure is likely to be an overestimate, it is a good habit to take note of the patient's case history, especially with regard to previous general anesthesias and related problems. The following should be examined: 1) mouth opening (>2.5-3 cm); 2) pharynx (Mallampati test); 3) jaw movement (i.e., the lower denture should be able to move forward of the upper one).

Measurements to be performed should include: 1) complete extension of the head over the neck with closed mouth [1]; 2) Patil distance should be more than 6 cm.

Radiological examinations are useful only in particular cases, such as laryngeal or tracheal deviations and stenosis. Anteroposterior and lateral projections are useful as well when a difficult intubation is predicted. CT and MRI provide better imaging and information. Of the easy and fast combinations of tests, Mallampati classification + Patil distance seem to have the highest sensitivity and specificity, i.e., with a higher incidence of true positives (sensitivity) and a lower incidence of false positives (specificity) [9].

Difficult intubation

The main rule to be followed is to prevent the consequences of a difficult intubation, such as hypoxia and bronchial inhalation. It is essential to achieve a facemask ventilation using 100% oxygen and to prevent bronchial inhalation (Sellick maneuver). When a satisfactory mask ventilation is obtained, any at-all-costs attempt to perform a tracheal intubation may provoke severe iatrogenic complications.

Knowledge of tracheal intubation techniques that offer alternatives to conventional direct laryngoscopy and airway management in the difficult and/or impossible intubation is an indispensable and peremptory requirement. At any rate, it is important to remember the correct use of straight blade and stylet, digital intubation, and oral or nasal blind intubation techniques. In addition, there are lightwands (Trachlight) which make blind tracheal intubation easier and devices which help oxygenate subjects that cannot be either intubated or ventilated with a facemask (LMA, Combitube, airway rapid access devices using direct approach or Seldingerís technique).

When the first intubation attempt fails, clinicians should ventilate the patient with 100% oxygen, make a note of the time, maintain an adequate anesthesia depth, check vital parameters, try to determine the problem, and resettle the equipment for airway management. Before going on with a second attempt, it is advisable for the clinician to be sure that sedation depth is adequate, to choose a smaller tube equipped with stylet, and to foresee the application of a BURP (backward, upward, and right-sided pressure) maneuver.

If the second attempt fails as well and intubation seems to be impossible, it will be necessary to oxygenate the patient, note the time, and ask for help. The following options should be absolutely taken into consideration: 1) postposing elective surgery; 2) placing a laryngeal mask to oxygenate the patient and resuming spontaneous ventilation. This option should be always considered in a difficult intubation emergency (see ASA algorithms [10]); 3) trying intubation through the LMA using a fiberoptic bronchoscope, which allows a direct view of the trachea and an intubation under direct view [11]; 4) trying intubation through the LMA using a lightwand without metal stylet, which allows transillumination of the cricoid membrane and semi-blind intubation of the trachea [12].

Once airway management has been achieved with the LMA, it may be impossible to accomplish an intubation through it using the above-mentioned techniques, either because the described instruments (fiberoptic scope, Trachlight) are not available or for anatomical reasons. Before going on with a third intubation attempt, it is necessary to check both vital parameters and the time since the first attempt; be sure that muscle tone is adequate for alignment of the three axes (mouth, pharynx, larynx).

If the instruments are available and clinicians are suitably trained, the third attempt should be carried out using the best-known and most adequate technique: Eschmann stylet, gum elastic bougie, lightwand, Bullard laryngoscope, fiberoptic bronchoscope intubation, or other special equipment. Of course, there is no reason not to try these techniques in a difficult intubation. If trained anesthesiologists make three unsuccessful attempts, they will have to resume spontaneous ventilation and postpone surgery.

In cases of emergency as well as when it is impossible to intubate and ventilate the patient, invasive methods should be used. Even if such emergencies are rare, it is necessary to be technically trained and to be well-equipped to deal with situations that threaten survival. A careful and codified clinical examination allows a difficult intubation to be predicted in 98% of cases, thus reducing the "surprise effect" of an unpredicted situation.

Fiberoptic intubation

Fiberoptic naso- or orotracheal intubation is certainly a first-choice technique in case of predicted difficult intubation, provided that the clinician is skilled in this field and that the fiberoptic scope used first. The alignment of the three axes is not required in fiberoptic intubation. This technique is effective when the clinician is very skilled and trained [13, 14]. Failures are rarely reported, provided that the contraindications to this technique are followed: bleeding, edema, large oropharyngo-laryngeal tumors, numerous previous attempts using other techniques with subsequent traumas, and, most importantly, an unskilled clinician. An emergency intubation is not an indication for fiberoptic laryngoscopy; on the contrary, according to some authors it is a contraindication. Ovassapian suggested a fiberoptic laryngoscopy technique in rapid sequence induction and intubation. Its main disadvantage is that the device is expensive and fragile. One cannot become a clinician skilled in fiberoptic laryngoscopy, for there is nothing in common between direct laryngoscopy and fiberoptic laryngoscopy, and self-learning is associated with a high incidence of failures [15] if without the guide of a skilled clinician. If spontaneous ventilation cannot be maintained – or the patient is in apnea – Patil mask [16] or endoscopy mask can be useful in ventilating the patient while intubating with the fiberoptic scope.

A technique associated with the LMA allows the patient to be safely ventilated in the intervals between one intubation attempt and the next and to facilitate fiberoptic maneuvers.

Thanks to a system of optic fibers, a Bullard laryngoscope [17] ensures a larynx view even without alignment of the three axes (oral, pharyngeal, laryngeal) and cervical rachis mobilization. Optic fibers run along the curved blade and allow illumination and view from the blade end. A working channel permits aspiration, oxygenation or administration of local anesthetics (lignocaine, etc.). This laryngoscope is particularly useful in cervical rachis traumas and pathologies because it does not call for mobilization. Use of a Bullard laryngoscope requires nearly the same training as for fiberoptic laryngoscopy [18]; it cannot replace the fiberoptic bronchoscopy in all cases, especially those involving limited mouth opening. A Bullard laryngoscope has the same disadvantages as the fiberoptic scope in cases of bleeding, abundant secretions, etc.

Laryngeal mask airway

The laryngeal mask airway (LMA), designed in 1981 by Brain, cannot be regarded as a new device in that it has been used in millions of placements in about 83 countries for years. Its guidelines include airway management during anesthesia of paralyzed or non paralyzed patients spontaneously breathing or under assisted ventilation. It plays an important part especially in predicted or unpredicted difficult intubation or while assisting breathing in cases of in- and outpatient emergency [19]. Use of the LMA is controversial in gastroesophageal junction pathology; upper abdominal surgery; and in the obese patient. But use of the LMA is absolutely contraindicated in full stomach and when high pressure insufflation is required to maintain airway management.

As an international reference center for the research on airway management with the LMA and prototypes, the University School Campus Bio-Medico, besides organizing theoretical–practical training courses in its application, has published two protocols ready for use in patients with predicted or unpredicted difficult intubations [20].

The long-discussed regurgitation problem is the reason why many clinicians distrust the LMA. In elective surgery fasted patients with no risk of regurgitation, the aspiration incidence – based on 547 publications until 1993 – is two out of 10 000 [21], comparable to that found for FM (facial mask) or TT (tracheal tube) ventilations (1.7 out of 10 000) [22, 23]. More recently, an incidence of 3.3% in patients in Trendelemburg or lithotomy positions [24], has been reported, while Verghese's 1996 publication describes three cases of regurgitation (0.03%), two of vomiting (0.017%), and one of gastric contents inhalation (0.009%) out of 11 910 anesthesias with the LMA [25]. As a result, the gastric laryngeal mask (GLM) [26, 27] has been developed and is being clinically tested. The GLM has a double access (laryngeal and esophageal) and one additional esophageal cuff. It allows a large gastric tube to be inserted through the additional lumen in order to withdraw gastric contents in an emergency patient who is probably unfasted.

Flexible or reinforced LMA

This is an LMA provided with a small reinforced, flexible and nondeformable tube. Its placement may be less smooth than that of the conventional LMA in the hands of an unskilled clinician, but it needs no accessory device, e.g., an introducer, if correctly inserted. The flexible LMA has been designed for head and neck surgeries where the conventional LMA tube may be too invasive or when it may be pressed or displaced during the surgical procedure. We have used it as a nasal LMA in dental surgery and have suggested a technique of retrograde placement [28, 29].

Unique

The Unique is a disposable LMA. This feature makes it especially suitable for emergencies (ambulance, out-patient first aid), or in cases of at-risk patients or those acknowledged to be positive to viral agents (hepatitis B, hepatitis C, HIV).

LMA Fastrach

The LMA Fastrach (LMA-FT) – sometimes also referred to as ILM (intubation laryngeal mask) – is a particular kind of LMA suitably designed for assisted ventilation and intubation in patients with high glottis. It has a rigid, curved silicone-coated metal structure and a single balancing bar instead of the common bars of the standard LMA. On the market since 1997, it is sold with a tube that facilitates intubation. This operation may be performed blind or associated with another technique, such as fiberoptic laryngoscopy or Trachlight without metal stylet, making it more successful. As any head extension is unnecessary to place the LMA-FT, it can be used to intubate patients at risk of cervical traumas; but it cannot be placed in patients with <2.5 cm mouth opening.

COPA

The COPA (cuffed oropharyngeal airway) is a device for airway management similar to a Guedel. It has a cuff at the pharyngeal end and a connector at the oral end, which allows it to be connected to common ventilation systems through a catheter mouth. COPA placement is the same as that of a common Guedel airway, with a rotatory movement but paying particular attention to rubbing of the cuff on the patientís teeth. It is indicated for patients spontaneously breathing or showing a reduced conscious state (pharmacological or pathological) so as to allow tolerance of the pharyngeal cuff.

Stylets

The stylet is a means to give stiffness to the tracheal tube in cases of slightly difficult intubations. It is about 30 cm long and is not hollow, as are introducers. Conventional stylets are made of metal while the latest ones are disposable and made of PVC or aluminum. The stylet lets the tip of the ETT (endotracheal tube) to stay curved (hockey stick-shaped) in order to allow sliding under the epiglottis even when the vocal folds are not perfectly visible. More recently, lightwands have been introduced. These add a transilluminating light to the standard intubation technique using a stylet, thereby permitting identification of the trachea.

Introducers

The introducer is a device that facilitates intubation in the case of Cormack grade 3 laryngoscopy, but it is not advisable for grade 4. Unlike stylets, introducers often have a hollow lumen and are over half a meter long. They can be more flexible as well as more rigid or reinforced, with a curved or linear tip. The softest ones are the tube exchangers, useful in replacing the ETT, i.e., as a tube exchanger in resuscitation. Real introducers, of which the best known is the gum elastic bougie, are used as a guide on which the tube can slide down to the trachea. The curved tip is slipped under the central part of the epiglottis and advanced for about 6 cm, until a typical click is heard on the tracheal rings or a stop on the carina is perceived. The tube is slipped down to the trachea on this guide. The hollow introducer can be connected to an oxygen source and a capnograph to oxygenate the patient and to evaluate exact placement before inserting the ETT. The ASA guidelines suggest the use of introducers in case of difficult intubation.

Hockey stick

The hockey stick is a particular kind of reusable stylet which facilitates a particularly high glottis intubation [30]. Its articulated structure allows bending of the

ETT tip to the angle chosen by simply manipulating it through its handle up to a 90° angle. Its main characteristic is that it allows one to change the ETT curve under laryngoscopic guide, as laryngeal structures are visible without manipulating the tube and may otherwise soiled with saliva or blood by using the hands. There are three sizes available: pediatric, teenage, and adult size.

Lighted stylets (lightwands)

The light-guided intubation of awake patients under topical anesthesia – or anaesthetized in spontaneous ventilation – is another approach to predicted difficult intubation. This simple, easy-to-learn, and rapid technique based on transillumination of the soft tissues is an improvement to blind nasotracheal intubation.

Trachlight

The Trachlight is a lightwand consisting of a handle, a wand provided with optic fiber, and a metal stylet. The lubricated wand is inserted inside a fitted ETT (not larger than 8 mm ID); the Trachlight tip must correspond to the end of the endotracheal tube. Its usage is based on the anatomical position of the trachea, anterior to the esophagus and subcutaneous.

The combination ETT-Trachlight is bent at 6-9 cm from the tip, forming an angle of about 90° (hockey stick-shaped). As the ETT tip passes over the tongue base and the epiglottis the soft tissues of the anterior neck will be illuminated; when there is an intense, well-defined, circumscribed glow level with the cricothyroid membrane, the ETT is in the laryngeal inlet. The light-guided tracheal intubation is a blind technique allowing tracheal intubation from the mouth or the nose. In fact, this procedure can rather be defined as a "semi-blind" technique because of the possibility to transilluminate and identify the anatomical landmarks. This technique can be learned in a short training course first, on a mannequin and then during elective surgery on normal-airway patients. Knowledge of the technique will improve its effectiveness and safety, even in the patient with predicted indexes of difficult intubation. Furthermore, the Trachlight allows tracheal intubation of patients with cervical column pathologies and/or a reduced mouth opening even at a severe degree, such as those wearing a halo collar [31], suffering from rheumatoid arthritis, or showing outcomes of facial traumas with temporomandibular joint ankylosis. The Trachlight allows nasal or oral intubation even of awake patients after topical anesthesia of the upper airway or in out-patient conditions, although the resuscitator cannot take his or her conventional position with respect to the patient.

Limitations to use of the Trachlight include the following: tumors, polyps, retropharyngeal abscess, infections, airway traumas, and foreign bodies.

Recent studies have pointed out that light-guided intubation is associated with fewer hemodynamic changes than conventional techniques using a laryngoscope

[32]. The use of the Trachlight without a metal stylet, in combination with standard LMA and LMA-FT, should be suggested for blind intubation. The Trachlight can also be used with conventional laryngoscopy in Cormack grade 3 difficult intubations.

Combined intubation techniques

These techniques make simultaneous use of more than one device for tracheal intubation, so as to increase the advantages and fill in the disadvantages of every single technique. Use of the LMA in combination with the Trachlight without metal stylet or with the fiberoptic bronchoscope is recommended to facilitate blind intubation through the conventional LMA or LMA-FT; alternatively, the Trachlight can be used with direct laryngoscopy in Cormack grade 3 cases [33]. Such combinations are especially indicated in difficult intubations or when the clinician is less skilled in using the individual techniques.

Blind nasotracheal intubation

In difficult intubations blind nasotracheal intubation was used as an alternative to laryngoscopy, before the introduction of fiberoptic laryngoscopy. It may be traumatic and cause hemorrhages and/or false submucous pathways and is not always successful, as it calls for extensive skill and experience, as any other technique does. With the patient conscious in spontaneous ventilation and sniffing position, blind nasotracheal intubation can be used in cases of limited mouth opening and when proper equipment or clinicians skilled in performing more sophisticated techniques are unavailable.

Retrograde intubation

This is a translaryngeal intubation guided by a small catheter or a suitable J-shaped guide. It is a relatively easy and quickly learned technique but calls for good anatomical knowledge and a certain degree of skill. It is mainly applied to awake patients under topical anesthesia with predicted difficult intubation, when conventional intubation attempts have failed. It may be used when it is impossible to see the vocal folds (blood, secretions, massive anatomical impairments) but never in emergency, as even those clinicians with skillful hands take some time to perform it [34].

Indications for retrograde intubation are: unstable cervical fractures, mandibular fractures, and anatomical abnormalities. Contraindications include: few anatomical landmarks (i.e., obesity), pretracheal masses (goiter), laryngotracheal pathologies (tumors, stenosis), hemorrhagic diatheses, and infections (i.e., paratracheal abscesses).

Technique

The patient is placed in a sniffing position with his neck extended; in patients with cervical pathologies, a neutral position is maintained.

The conventional technique requires cricothyroid puncture. The cricothyroid membrane is a nonvascularized structure which provides good access without any bleeding risk. However, the distance (1 cm) between the puncture area and the vocal folds may cause the ETT to take a too acute angle, making sliding of the tube into the trachea harder. Puncture at the cricotracheal ligament level may be more advantageous because the greater distance between the inlet and the vocal folds allows easier placement of the ETT, but involves a higher risk of bleeding. A guide catheter is removed from the nose or the mouth and then passed through the needle inserted in the trachea and the ETT is slipped over it.

Technique-related complication may be esophageal perforation, hemoptysis, tracheal hematoma with distal obstruction, laryngeal edema, laryngospasm, vocal folds lesions, tracheitis, and pretracheal infection.

Upper airway anesthesia avoids sympathetic reflexes and laryngospasm. Most commonly use is: 1) 4 ml 2% lignocaine for the translaryngeal puncture at cricothyroid membrane level (mct); 2) supplement of hypopharyngeal and pharyngeal anesthesia with 10% xylocaine spray. There are special retrograde intubation sets; if these are not available, common peridural or central vein sets can be used.

Suggestions for predicted difficult intubation

1. The patient must be awake.
2. If topical anesthesia and sedation are performed it will be always necessary to maintain spontaneous ventilation.
3. An adequate system of monitoring the patient, i.e., saturation measurement device; arterial pressure, ECG, capnograph, is always needed.
4. Prior to any intubation attempt the patient needs to be preoxygenated; 100% oxygen over a period of 60 s with full vital capacity breaths allows the patient to tolerate apnea for 8 min without developing any hypoxia [35].
5. In borderline patients with predicted difficult intubation risks, it is suggested to use short-action paralyzing drugs together with general anesthetics whose effects are not excessively depressive over ventilation.

Suggestions for unpredicted difficult intubation

1. The patient should be routinely preoxygenated in order to have enough time to call for help and arrange the necessary techniques.
2. The patient's oxymetry, ECG, and capnography should always be monitored.
3. Tracheal inhalation should be prevented through a Sellick maneuver.
4. A failed intubation should be immediately recognized.

5. Intubation attempts – up to three – are to be suspended to let the patient be oxygenated with a facemask or with the aid of a laryngeal mask.
6. A good sedation depth should be maintained to avoid laryngeal spasm.
7. Techniques that may worsen a regional edema, which hampers mask ventilation and a possible fiberoptic laryngoscopy, should not be used.

"Cannot intubate, cannot ventilate" situations

This event more often occurs when adequate equipment is not available; in patients with mouth or nose anatomical abnormalities, in those with thick beards, obesity, and airway obstruction; edentulous and asthmatic patients; those suffering from pneumothorax or massive pleural effusion; and in patients who cannot be intubated and risk laryngospasm on waking up from anesthesia and myoresolution.

The Combitube

The Combitube can be useful in the "cannot intubate, cannot ventilate" situation. It is a double-lumen and double-cuffed tube intended to be inserted blindly from the mouth. The esophageal lumen is blind at the distal end but has eight perforations that are located at the level of the lower pharynx. The tracheal lumen is open at the distal end and unperforated throughout. When the distal lumen is into the esophagus, ventilation is performed through the perforations on the wall of the esophageal lumen. While the distal cuff prevents aspiration of a possible regurgitation, the proximal cuff avoids any air leakage from the mouth. When ventilation is through the trachea, correct placement will be confirmed by bilateral auscultation and capnography. The distal cuff acts like that of a conventional ETT. Gastric or esophageal ruptures have been described as complications associated with placement of the Combitube into the esophagus [36]. Glottic obstruction may occur if the Combitube is inserted too deeply or the proximal cuff overinflated. The Combitube is especially useful when the neck cannot – or should not – be extended. It has been included in the latest ASA guidelines for difficult airway management and in the "Guidelines for Cardiopulmonary Resuscitation and Emergency Cardiac Care" of the American Heart Association [37]. It has also been recommended in obstetric patients, who cannot be intubated or mask-ventilated, and especially in obese patients [38]. Recent studies confirm its value during CPR [39, 40].

Since the Combitube can be inserted without the help of a laryngoscope, airway management is not hampered by either adverse environmental factors or staff unskilled in the use of a laryngoscope [41]. In patients with massive bleeding or continued vomiting, a failed view of the vocal folds is no longer an obstacle to intubation. This is the major indication for use of the Combitube by anesthesiologists, besides its suitability in patients with difficult anatomical situations. Gastric fluids can be suctioned through the tracheal lumen when the tube is in the esophagus. The oropharyngeal balloon protects the airway and effectively prevents aspiration of any oral contents. The Combitube is, however, contraindicated in patients shorter than 5 feet; patients with intact gag reflexes; patients with known esophageal pathologies; patients with obstruction of the upper airways, etc.

Transtracheal jet ventilation

This is a simple technique that can ensure an adequate oxygenation for survival under emergency conditions, when it is impossible to intubate and ventilate the patient. In the case of a worsening hypoxia it ensures 100% oxygen minimum ventilation using a short catheter (peripheral venous catheter) placed into the trachea. Transtracheal oxygenation provides the time needed to perform intubation using another technique, i.e., fiberoptic laryngoscopy, lightwand, or Bullard laryngoscope. The larger the catheter, the more important the tidal volume administered; as it will improve hypoxia, yet is not sufficient to reduce hypercapnia. Intercricoid membrane puncture is usually performed with a 14-gauge short intravenous cannula which is directed downward into the tracheal lumen. With the cannula inserted, if the necessary equipment is available, a high-frequency jet ventilation can be used, balloon ventilation being not very effective. Alternatively, it is possible to perform a manual jet ventilation using a high-flow oxygen source.

Equipment

To perform transtracheal jet ventilation (TTJV) the following equipment is needed:
1. high-pressure O_2 source (>50 psi–1 psi=70 cm H_2O);
2. rigid connection circuit;
3. 16-12-gauge transtracheal catheter.

When the cricothyroid membrane is seen with the head extended (if possible), a 12-14-gauge catheter is connected to a 20 ml syringe. The catheter is held like a pen and, with the tip of the needle turned caudally forming a 45° angle, a puncture is made level with the cricothyroid membrane. Air aspiration confirms catheter correct placement. Then, the O_2 source is connected through the proper Luer lock connection or by connecting the catheter to a pediatric tube connector.

Note that TTJV should be performed in desperate situations only and when all other techniques have failed. Benumof suggests that TTJV should be used in desperate situations in patients with a distorted airway anatomy. Such advice calls seriously for questioning use of this procedure. More conservative approaches, such as percutaneous cricothyrotomy followed by manual ventilation, are surely more advisable under these circumstances.

The TTJV may be very useful in the case of an obese patient when intubation or ventilation is impossible. This situation usually needs a high-pressure inspiratory peak in order to give at least an acceptable ventilation, which might be impossible even performing a four-hand mask ventilation.

Cricothyrotomy

Cricothyrotomy is a technique able to supply an airway access between the lower margin of the thyroid cartilage and the upper end of the cricoid cartilage. This area is the most easily approachable of the subglottic respiratory tree [42]. The technique is indicated for: severe maxillofacial trauma; cervical column deformity at a severe degree; temporomandibular ankylosis (rheumatoid arthritis); laryngotracheal trauma due to repeated attempts of tracheal intubation with complete airway obstruction; hypopharyngeal burn; mechanical obstruction; presence of foreign bodies.

Cricothyrotomy allows quicker oxygenation and ventilation than conventional tracheotomy, which cannot be performed easily under emergency conditions. It is an elective maneuver for survival when the patient cannot be intubated and ventilated. In case of impossible tracheal intubation with complete obstruction, it allows airway management and maintenance rapidly and easily.

Technique and anatomy

A transversal cut is made between the two anatomical landmarks – the lower margin of the thyroid cartilage and the upper margin of the cricoid cartilage. The cricothyroid artery may cross the cricothyroid membrane and cause bleeding, which needs to be sutured or electrocoagulated. The cannula can be placed using two techniques and sets: 1) Seldinger system, Minitrach II Melker; and 2) direct procedure system, Minitrach I Ravussin Patil Tracheoquick.

Tracheotomy

Tracheotomy is a particularly dangerous technique, to be performed under emergency conditions when the patient is hypoxic. It calls for skilled clinicians who will not compromise the future functional prognosis. When possible, it should be carried out in awake patients, under topical anesthesia, or after the insertion of a transtracheal catheter and a jet ventilation.

Conclusions

Emergency airway management is far more difficult in out-patient situations. In these cases awake intubation is the elective treatment and, when a sedation is needed, it should be performed with the patient spontaneously breathing. In hospitalized patients, in case of predicted difficult intubation, fiberoptic laryngoscopy is still the reference method. Under unpredicted conditions, mask ventilation or intercricoid ventilation avoids the onset of hypoxia. To oxygenate the patient, the laryngeal mask, the Combitube, and transtracheal ventilation can be alternatives to intubation. Thus, it is necessary to teach the different techniques, which are complementary rather than alternative. Theoretical, and especially practical, teaching of noninvasive techniques is to be carried out on mannequins, animals, and/or cadavers, or in elective surgery. Self-learning, or trying out a poorly known technique, should obviously be avoided in emergency situations.

References

1. Bellhouse CP, Doré C (1988) Criteria for estimating likelihood of difficulty of tracheal intubation with the Macintosh laryngoscope. Anaesth and Inten Care 16:329-337
2. Aro L, Takki S, Aroma U (1971) Technique for difficult intubation. Br J Anaesth 43:1081-1083
3. Crinquette V, Vilette B, Solanet C et al (1991) Utilisation du PVC, laryngoscope pour intubation difficile. Ann Fr Anesth Réanim 10:589-594
4. Samsoon GLT, Young JRB (1987) Difficult tracheal intubation: a retrospective study Anaesth 42:487-490
5. Benumof JL (1995) Foreword. Anaesth Clin NA 13:2
6. American Society of Anesthesiologists Committee on Professional Liability (1988) Preliminary study in closed claims. ASA Newsletter 52(4):8-10
7. Cormack RS, Lehane J (1984) Difficult intubation in obstetrics. Anaesth 39:1105-1111
8. Norton ML, Brown ACD (1991) Atlas of the difficult airway: a source book. Mosby, St Louis
9. Frerk C (1991) Predicting difficult intubation. Anaesth 46:1005
10. American Society of Anesthesiologists Task Force on Management of the Difficult Airway (1993) Practice guidelines for difficult airway. 78:597-602
11. Smith JE, Sherwood NA (1991) Combined use of laryngeal mask airway and fiberoptic laryngoscope in difficult intubation. Anaesth Intens Care 19:471-472
12. Morelli A, Cataldo R, Marchionni L et al (1997) Trachlight senza guida metallica per intubazione tracheale attraverso LMA: dati preliminari. Min Anestesiol 63(Suppl 2)9:97
13. Ovassapian A, Yelich SJ, Dykes MHM, Golman ME (1989) Learning fiberoptic intubation: use of simulators vs traditional teaching. Br J Anaesth 61:217-220
14. Vaugham RS (1991) Training in fiberoptic laryngoscopy. Br J Anaesth 66:538-540
15. Dykes MHM, Ovassapian A (1989) Dissemination of fiberoptic airway endoscopy skills by means of a workshop utilizing models. Br J Anaesth 63:595-597
16. Patil V, Stehling LC, Zauder HL, Koch JP (1982) Mechanical aids for fiberoptic endoscopy. Anesthesiol 57:69-70
17. Saunders PA, Giesecke AH (1989) Clinical assessment of the adult Bullard laryngoscope. Canad J Anesth 36:118-119
18. Dyson A, Harris J, Bhatia K (1990) Rapidity and accuracy of tracheal intubation in a mannequin: comparison of the fiberoptic with the Bullard laryngoscope. Br J Anaesth 65:268-270
19. Brain AIJ (1991) Prehospital and disaster medicine. 7th World Congress on or Emergency and Disaster Medicine. (Abstract) pp 254
20. Agrò F (1996) Maschera laringea: indicazioni e prospettive di applicazione. Min Anestesiol 62(Suppl 1)9:686-99
21. Brimacombe J, Berry A (1995) The incidence of aspiration associated with the laryngeal mask airway: a meta analysis of published literature. J Clin Anaesth 7:297-305
22. Brimacombe J, Berry A (1996) Incidence of aspiration with the laryngeal mask airway. Anaesthesiol Abstract Book 605:1272
23. Kallar SK (1988) Aspiration pneumonitis: fact or fiction? Probl Anesth 2:29-36
24. El Mikatti N, Luthra AD, Healy EJ, Mortimer AJ (1995) Gastric regurgitation during general anaesthesia in different positions with the laryngeal mask airway. Anaesth 50:12

25. Verghese C, Brimacombe J (1996) Survey of laryngeal mask airway usage in 11910 patients: safety and efficacy for conventional and non conventional usage. Anesth Analg 82:129-133
26. Brain AIJ, Verghese C, Strube P, Brimacombe J (1995) A new laryngeal mask prototype. Anaesth 50:42-48
27. Agrò F, Brain A, Gabbrielli A et al (1997) Prevention of tracheal aspiration in a patient with a high risk of regurgitation using a new double-lumen gastric laryngeal mask airway. Gastr Endos 46-3:257-258
28. Agrò F, Marchionni L, De Ponte FS, Favaro R, Carassiti M, Cataldo R (1998) Campus Bio-Medico technique for nasolaryngeal ventilation with reinforced laryngeal mask in dental surgery: a patient report. J Craniofacial Surg (in press)
29. Marchionni L, Agrò F, Favaro R, Verghese C, Brimacombe J (1997) The flexible laryngeal mask as a nasal airway. Anaesth Analg 85(5):1179
30. Picarazzi A, Cataldo R, Morelli A, Baldelli L, Agrò F (1997) Utilizzo dell'Hockey Stick nell'intubazione oro-tracheale: dati preliminari. Min Anestesiol 63(Suppl 2)9:98
31. Cataldo R, Marchionni L, Carassiti M, Agrò F (1997) Intubazione tracheale con Trachlight in un caso di instabilità cervicale. Min Anestesiol 63(Suppl 2)9:97
32. Hung OR, Pytka S, Murphy MF et al (1995) Clinical trial of a new lightwand to intubate the trachea. Anesthesiol 42(9):826-830
33. Agrò F, Brimacombe J, Carassiti M, Morelli A, Giampalmo M, Cataldo R (1998) Lighted style T as an aid to blind tracheal intubation the LMA (Letter). J Clin Anesth 10(3):263-264
34. Sanchez A, Pallares V (1995) Retrograde intubation technique. In: Benumof JL (ed) Airway Management. Mosby, St Louis, pp 320-341
35. Veroli PH, Samii K (1990) À propos de la préoxygénation avant intubation difficile. Ann Fr Anesth Réanim 9:569
36. Johnson KR, Genovesi MG, Lassar KH (1976) Esophageal obturator airway: use and complications. J Am Soc Emerg Phis 5:36
37. Guidelines for Cadiopulmonary resuscitation and emergency cardiac care (1992) Recommendations of the 1992 national Conference of the American Heart Association. JAMA 268:2203
38. Wissler RN (1993) The esophageal-tracheal Combitube. Anesthesiol Rev 20:147-152
39. Rumball CJ, MacDonald D (1997) The PTL, Combitube, laryngeal mask and oral airway: a randomized prehospital comparative study of ventilatory device effectiveness and cost-effectiveness in 470 cases of cardiorespiratory arrest. Prehosp Emerg Care 1:1-10
40. Vezina D, Lessard MR, Bussiéres J, Topping C, Trépanier CA (1998) Complication associated with the use of the Esophageal-Tracheal Combitube. Can J Anaesth 45:76-80
41. Johnson JC, Atherton GL (1991) The esophageal tracheal Combitube: an alternate route to airway management. JEMS 29:3
42. Melker JR, Orlando GFJ (1996) Percutaneous dilational cricothyrotomy and tracheotomy. In: Benumof JL (ed) Airway Management. Mosby, St Louis, pp 484-312

Chapter 11

Thermal homeostasis in trauma patients

M.E. Crawford, H. Rask

Evolution and thermoregulation

Thermoregulatory mechanisms and controls are relatively recent from an evolutionary standpoint as animals have either recruited or modified other regulatory systems [1]. Consequently, body temperature control is not an isolated regulated system in vertebrates but more a hierarchically integrated multiple system.

The pineal gland is known to transduce environmental information for photoperiodic and seasonal adjustments to the preoptic area of the anterior hypothalamus via its primary secretory hormone melanin. The hypothalamus integrates the information and then sets the effector recruitment for each control system consistent with the metabolic rate of the animal.

Physiology

The temperature of the body is regulated almost entirely by nervous feedback mechanisms operating through temperature-regulating centers located in the hypothalamus. There are four mechanisms of heat loss from the body:
- electromagnetic radiation;
- convection;
- conduction;
- evaporation.

In general, in dry air, the nude body is capable of maintaining a normal body core temperature between 36.1°C and 37.7°C. For these feedback mechanisms to operate, detectors must exist in the peripheral as well as in the central nervous system.

The principal area in the brain in which heat from a thermode affects body temperature control consists of the preoptic and anterior hypothalamic nucleus of the hypothalamus where large numbers of heat-sensitive neurons and about a third as many cold-sensitive neurons function as temperature sensors and increase the firing rate as body temperature either rises or falls.

When the preoptic area is heated, the skin immediately breaks out into profuse sweating while at the same time the skin blood vessels over the entire body become greatly vasodilated. In addition, excess body heat production is inhibited [1].

The skin is endowed with both cold and warmth receptors with a distribution factor of 10:1 and, therefore, peripheral detection of temperature mainly concerns detecting cool and cold instead of warm temperatures [2, 3].

When skin is chilled over the entire body, immediate reflex effects are invoked to increase the temperature of the body by providing a strong stimulus to cause shivering, with a resultant increase in the rate of body heat production, by inhibiting the process of sweating and by promoting skin vasoconstriction to diminish the transfer of body heat to the skin.

The posterior hypothalamus plays a major role in integrating peripheral and central temperature signals.

The most important heat-conserving feature is the number of active measures carried out whenever the perception of coldness becomes a conscious one. These may include insulation via clothing and physical activity, with a capacity of increasing the basal metabolic rate 20-fold.

Temperature decreasing mechanisms consist of:
- vasodilatation mediated by sympathetic centres in the posterior hypo- thalamus where the skin heat transfer rate increases eightfold;
- sweating with tenfold removal of the basal rate of body heat production;
- decrease in heat production with inhibition of shivering and chemical thermo- genesis;
- voluntary acts (exposure).

Temperature increasing mechanisms consist of:
- skin vasoconstriction throughout the body caused by posterior hypo-thalamic sympathetic centres;
- piloerection caused by sympathetic nervous stimulation;
- increase in heat production by shivering;
- sympathetic excitation of heat production;
- thyroxine secretion;
- voluntary acts (clothing and physical activity).

The primary motor centre for shivering is located in the dorsomedial portion of the posterior hypothalamus near the wall of the third ventricle where signals increase the tone of the skeletal muscles throughout the body. Shivering begins whenever the tone rises above a critical level.

The degree of chemical thermogenesis is proportionate to the amount of brown fat in the tissues containing large numbers of mitochondriae where uncoupled oxidation occurs. In adult human beings who have almost no brown fat, heat production seldom increases more than 15%. Infants have small amounts of brown fat in the interscapular space and heat production may be increased by as much as 100%.

Increased thyroxin levels increase metabolism in general and exposure to cold surroundings for several weeks may lead to enlargement of the thyroid gland.

Thermal regulation in children

Thermoregulation during exposure to hot or cold environments differs between children and adults. Children have a much higher surface area to mass ratio, allowing more dry heat loss and less evaporative cooling in warm conditions; however, extreme conditions hot or cold, result in a higher rate of heat absorption and heat loss, respectively. The lower body fat in girls than in women offers less insulation and the smaller blood volume may limit the potential for heat transfer during heat exposure and compromise exercise performance in the heat [4]. The main physiological difference between children and adults lies in the sweating mechanism. This affects their thermoregulation during heat exposure due to a lower sweating rate per gland and not to a lower number of glands. The higher metabolic cost of locomotion in children provides an added strain on the thermoregulatory system during exercise in the heat but may prove advantageous during acute cold exposure by increasing heat production. In boys, lower haemoglobin concentrations and cardiac output levels during exercise may increase cardiovascular strain in the heat as compared to conditions in adult men.

The effectiveness of thermoregulation is reflected by the stability of core temperature and children are characterized by a higher skin temperature but similar rectal temperature in neutral temperature conditions. Temperatures are higher than in adults while walking and running. In cold conditions skin temperatures are lower due to higher degrees of vasoconstriction.

Temperature monitoring

Measurement of body core temperature values may be performed at various sites well-known to the clinician; however, traditionally, rectal recordings are used routinely. When comparing brain temperature (ventriculostomy catheter) with bladder and rectal temperatures in head-injury patients, Henker et al. demonstrated that brain values usually were greater than bladder and rectal values [5] with standard deviations of the difference ranging from 0.30°C-0.80°C between brain and bladder and 0.32°C-1.08°C between brain and rectum. In the majority of patients differences were greater at temperatures outside the normal temperature range and it was concluded that bladder- and rectal temperatures often underrepresent brain temperatures following traumatic injury, particularly when the patient is hypo- or hyperthermic.

Mild to moderate levels of hypothermia may profoundly reduce the histological and biochemical sequelae of cerebral ischaemic injury and therefore monitoring of the exact brain temperature seems to be essential when dealing with trauma victims. Watts, in 1998 [6], studied 112 trauma patients and found that, at core temperatures of less than 34°C hypothermic coagulopathy was due to decreased platelet function and enzyme activity slowing, whereas at core temperatures above 34°C, there was a significant hypercoagulability.

Animal studies indicate [7] that:
- brain injury itself does not influence brain temperature;
- anaesthesia alone decreases brain temperature to levels producing cerebral protection;
- external monitoring of the temporalis muscle temperature may provide a reliable indirect measure of brain temperature following brain injury.

Hyperthermia and ischemic brain injury

Moderate elevations of brain temperature, when present during or after ischaemia, may markedly worsen the resulting injury. In standardized models of transient forebrain ischaemia, intra-ischaemic brain temperature elevations to 39°C enhance and accelerate severe neuropathological alterations in vulnerable brain regions and induce damage to structures not ordinarily affected. The action of otherwise neuroprotective drugs in ischaemia may be nullified by mild hyperthermia and, even with a delay of 24 h after an acute insult pathological and neurobehavioural outcome can be worsened [8].

Mechanisms are:
– enhanced release of neurotransmitters;
– exaggerated oxygen radical production;
– more extensive blood-brain barrier breakdown;
– increased numbers of potentially damaging ischaemic depolarizations in the focal ischemic penumbra;
– impaired recovery of energy metabolism;
– enhanced inhibition of protein kinases;
– worsening of cytoskeletal proteolysis.

Hypothermia and neuroprotection

Profound whole-body hypothermia, typically carried out in conjunction with extracorporeal bypass, has long been employed during cardiac and neurosurgical procedures. More recently, studies in small animal experimental models of cerebral ischaemia have provided evidence that even small decreases in brain temperature confer striking protection against ischaemic neuronal injury. Hypothermia retards the rate of high-energy phosphate depletion during ischaemia and promotes postischaemic metabolic recovery [9]. Mild intra-ischaemic hypothermia markedly attenuates the release of glutamate into the extracellular space of the brain and significantly diminishes the release of dopamine. The inhibition of calcium-calmodulin dependent protein kinase II triggered by normothermic ischaemia is prevented by hypothermia, as is the translocation and inhibition of the key regulatory enzyme protein kinase C. Hypothermia also seems to facilitate the resynthesis of ubiquitin following ischaemia.

In the setting of focal cerebral ischaemia moderate brain hypothermia reduces the infarct size and papers on "pharmacoprotection" may falsely have attributed these neuroprotective properties to the drug induced hypothermia.

Trauma and thermoregulation

In trauma, the normal thermoregulatory mechanisms are often compromised and hypothermia is reported to be present approximately in half of all major trauma cases (42%-66%) and has been associated with increased mortality rate in patients stratified by anatomic indices of injury severity [10, 11].

There are several factors causing hypothermia in trauma patients, some pertaining to the injury itself and some to treatment- and other procedures: head injuries may compromise central regulatory mechanisms, heat production and conservation via voluntary actions are eliminated, controlled ventilation increases heat loss, anaesthetics lead to peripheral vasodilatation, heat loss is increased due to convection, radiation and evaporation.

Early post-traumatic hypothermia has been found to correlate with physiological indicators of volume deficit, independently of the amount of intravenous fluid received [12] whereas no connection was observed between admission core temperature and time from injury, blood alcohol level, or presence of severe closed head injury. Hypothermic patients ($<35°C$) had a lower predicted probability of survival and a higher mortality rate than euthermic patients, however, when patients were stratified by physiological and anatomical indicators of injury severity, mortality rates among the euthermic and hypothermic patients were not significantly different.

In a randomized prospective trial including 57 hypothermic critically injured patients requiring a pulmonary artery catheter and randomized to a rapid rewarming protocol using continuous arteriovenous rewarming (CAVR) or standard rewarming, it was demonstrated that the patients treated with CAVR had significantly less early mortality and lower fluid volume requirements [13].

Various adverse effects of hypothermia have been reported in trauma patients including increased mortality [11, 13, 14] and compromised coagulation [6].

Hypercapnia, which may be encountered during diving operations or by patients under general anaesthesia with spontaneous respiration, alters the basis thermoregulatory responses [15]. In cold-exposed animals, 3%-10% inspired CO_2 impairs thermal homeostasis by attenuating shivering and promoting heat loss through peripheral vasodilatation.

Maintenance of normothermia

Mechanisms responsible for the cardiovascular manifestations of hypothermia remain unclear and are based in the relationship between brain temperature, neuroendocrine response and resulting vascular refelex mechanisms. In a randomized prospective study of 300 patients undergoing thoracic or vascular surgery and who had documented coronary artery disease, the relative risk of morbid cardiac events was calculated and outcome assessed in a double-blind fashion in a hypo- and normothermic group [16]. Hypothermia was an independent predictor of cardiac morbidity and risk was reduced by 55% when normothermia was maintained. Other studies demonstrate that maintaining core normothermia decreases the duration of postanaesthetic recovery [17].

Several techniques are available for rewarming procedures ranging from passive heat retention by manipulation of surrounding atmosphere and by low flow anaesthesia systems, to additional thermal insulation by reflective or heated blankets, to forced-air warming and a number of invasive or semi-invasive warming procedures. Comparison of these techniques in connection with major surgical procedures indicate that passive heat retention is ineffective in maintaining intraoperative normothermia and definitely inferior to active forced-air warming [18].

Although forced-air warming rapidly increases intraoperative core temperatures, it is reportedly ineffective postoperatively. A major difference between these two periods is that arteriovenous shunts are usually dilated during surgery, whereas vasoconstriction is uniform in hypothermic postoperative patients [19]. Vasoconstriction may decrease efficacy of warming because its major physiological purposes are to reduce cutaneous heat transfer and restrict heat transfer between the two thermal compartments. Differences between intra- and postoperative conditions also result from nonthermoregulatory anaesthetic-induced vasodilatation.

Future aspects

Thermal effects on the body may be simulated with computer technology. In an American study on the effect of application of aircraft cabin water spray systems, temperature changes were computed at 25 body segments in response to water immersion, cold-air exposure, and windy conditions [20]. Inputs to the temperature controller were: a) temperature change signals from skin segments; and b) integrated signal of the product of skin and head-core (hypothalamic) temperature changes. The controller-simulated changes in blood flow to skin and muscle and heat production by shivering. Two controller parameters were adjusted to obtain good predictions of temperature and heat production experimental data in head-out, water immersion (0°C-28°C) studies in humans.

In a similar Japanese study, a computer program was developed for the numerical analysis of thermal conditions in which a cylindrical model consisting of internal multi-layers formed the basis of a linear combination of the modified Bessel functions [21] and internal tissue temperatures, heat fluxes and blood temperatures of the thigh, crus and foot segments were calculated. With this algorithm, utilizing the new heat transfer equation, it was possible to demonstrate characteristics of each segment of the human body.

References

1. Kowal-Vern A, Sharp-Pucci MM, Walenga JM, Dries DJ, Gamelli RL (1996) Thermoregulatory spectrum in vertebrates. Indian J Exp Biol 44(2):1053-1070
2. Guyton AC (1991) Basic neuroscience, 2nd ed. WB Saunders, Philadelphia, pp 360-364
3. Boulant JA, Dean JB (1986) Temperature receptors in the central nervous system. Annu Rev Physiol 48:39
4. Falk B (1998) Effects of thermal stress during rest and exercise in the paediatric population. Sports Med 25(4):221-240
5. Henker RA, Brown SD, Marion DW (1998) Comparison of brain temperature with bladder and rectal temperatures in adults with severe head injury. Neurosurgery 42(5):1071-1075

6. Watts DD, Trask A, Soeken K, Perdue P, Dols S, Kaufmann C (1998) Hypothermic coagulopathy in trauma: effect of varying levels of hypothermia on enzyme speed, platelet function, and fibrinolytic activity. J Trauma 44(5):846-854

7. Jiang JY, Lyeth BG, Clifton GL, Jenkins LW, Hamm RJ, Hayes RL (1991) Relationship between body and brain temperature in traumatically brain-injured rodents. J Neurosurg 74(3):492-496

8. Ginsberg MD, Busto R (1998) Combating hyperthermia in acute stroke: a significant clinical concern. Stroke 29(2):529-534

9. Ginsberg MD, Sternau LL, Globus MY, Dietrich WD, Busto R (1992) Therapeutic modulation of brain temperature: relevance to ischaemic brain injury. Cerebrovasc Brain Metab Rev 4(3):189-225

10. Luna GK, Maier RV, Pavlin EG, Anardi D, Copass MK, Oreskovich MR (1987) Incidence and effect of hypothermia in seriously injured patients. J Trauma 27(9):1014-1018

11. Jurkovich GJ, Greiser WB, Luterman A, Curreri PW (1987) Hypothermia in trauma victims: an ominous predictor of survival. J Trauma 27(9):1019-1024

12. Steinemann S, Shackford SR, Davis JW (1990) Implications of admission hypothermia in trauma patients. J Trauma 42(2):200-202

13. Gentilello LM, Jurkovich GJ, Stark MS, Hassantash SA, O`Keefe GE (1997) Is hypothermia in the victim of major trauma protective or harmful? A randomized, prospective study. Ann Surg 44(4):439-447

14. Gentilello LM, Cobean RA, Offner PJ, Soderberg RW, Jurkovich GJ (1992) Continuous arteriovenous rewarming: rapid reversal of hypothermia in critically ill patients. J Trauma 226(3):316-325

15. Johnston CE, Elias DA, Ready AE, Giesbrecht GG (1996) Hypercapnia lowers the shivering threshold and increases core cooling rate in humans. Aviat Space Environ Med 44(2):438-444

16. Frank SM, Fleisher LA, Breslow MJ, Higgins MS, Olson KF, Kelly S, Beattie C (1997) Perioperative maintenance of normothermia reduces the incidence of morbid cardiac events. JAMA 277(14):1127-1134

17. Lenhardt R, Marker E, Goll V, Tschernich H, Kurz A, Sessler DI, Narzt E, Lackner F (1997) Mild intraoperative hypothermia prolongs postanaesthetic recovery. Anesthesiology 277(14):1318-1323

18. Berti M, Casati A, Torri G, Aldegheri G, Lugani D, Fanelli G (1997) Active warming, not passive heat retention, maintains normothermia during combined epidural-general anesthesia for hip and knee arthroplasty. J Clin Anesth 9(6):482-486

19. Clough D, Kurz A, Sessler DI, Christensen R, Xiong J (1996) Thermoregulatory vasoconstriction does not impede core warming during cutaneous heating. Anesthesiology 85(2):281-288

20. Wolf MB, Garner RP (1997) Simulation of human thermoregulation during water immersion: application to an aircraft cabin water-spray system. Ann Biomed Eng 25(4):620-634

21. Yokoyama S, Kakuta N, Ochifuji K (1997) Development of a new algorithm for heat transfer equation in the human body and its applications. Appl Human Sci 16(4):153-159

Chapter 12

Prevention and management of pulmonary inhalation

M.E. Crawford, H. Rask

An increasing number of thermal injuries are encountered worldwide due to technological progress in the commercial industry as well as political warfare. In the USA, more than 2 million people require medical attention every year, leading to 500 000 emergency ward visits and 70 000 hospital admissions, of which 20 000 are transferred to a specialized burns unit [1, 2]. Thermal injuries result in 9 000 fatal cases annually. In Denmark, the incidence of thermal burns is approximately 1 per 100 per year, i.e. 50 000 cases, of which 150 are severe with involvement of more than 20% body surface area (personal communication).

Inhalation lesions are the most frequent factors responsible for mortality (approx. 75%) in patients suffering from thermal injury where primary evaluation of the patient with focus on thermal injury and / or toxin inhalation is essential for outcome [3-5]. Carbon monoxide and other toxic products of combustion are major determinants of severity and early hypoxaemia contributes to over 50% of deaths. In many areas of the world paraffin flames predominate [6] over all the aetiological agents of inhalation injury, the toxic agents being:
– hydrogen cyanide;
– hydrogen fluoride;
– hydrogen chloride;
– nitrogen oxides;
– sulphur dioxide;
– ammonia;
– acrolein.

Hydrogen cyanide gas, the most toxic product of combustion [7], is released from synthetic polymers in building materials and furnishing and was reported to be present in four of six fatalities in Ohio [8].

Smoke inhalation affects all levels of the respiratory system and the degree of injury depends on duration, exposure level, fume temperature and toxicity, concentration and solubility of toxic gases, closed space entrapment and pre-existing diseases. Clinical signs are hoarseness, altered voice, wheezing, coughing, stridor, dyspnoea, carbonaceous sputum, disorientation, and often singed facial and nasal hairs [1]. Endoscopy or the presence of carbon monoxide haemoglobin confirms the diagnosis.

Demographics

Demographics reveal (1985-1991; New Jersey; n=727) disproportionate percentages of children younger than 11 years and elderly persons older than 70 years, males with smoking materials as most common source and maximum risk during the night [9, 10, 28]. Risk factors for smoke-related morbidity as identified following the World Trade Center bombing disaster [11] are:
– increased age;
– presence of pre-existing cardiopulmonary condition;
– entrapment in a confined space (elevator);
– prolonged evacuation time.

Pathophysiological mechanisms

The upper airways have a large heat exchange capacity and heat damage is often confined to this area, resulting in rapidly developing oedema. Lower airway damage is caused by chemical and particle irritation and is followed by mucosal damage, local and systemic inflammatory response and capillary leak [8].

Smoke inhalation results in a decrease in lung compliance, severe airway inflammation, mucosal sloughing, atelectasis formation, increase in lung water and alveolar oedema. Animal studies utilizing particle filtering techniques and shunting fractions conclude that the injury is cased by the particle phase and not the gas phase [12].

Toxic inhalants cause injury through a variety of different mechanisms, including direct irritation of the respiratory tract mucosa, asphyxiation, and systemic absorption of the toxin. The nature and extent of the acute injury depends on the inhalant´s water solubility, aerodynamic features, pH and concentration. Phosgene inhalation causes a severe non-cardiogenic pulmonary oedema characterized by an influx of neutrophils into the lung, and animal studies seem to suggest that impairing leucocyte migration and the generation of the chemotaxin leukotriene B4 with the microtubular poison colchicine, significantly reduces neutrophil influx, lung injury, and mortality [14]. As activated neutrophils extrude cytotoxic proteases, serine protease inhibititors (gabexate mesilate) also may attenuate the degradation in microvascular integrity associated with smoke inhalation injury [29].

Smoke inhalation is a particularly challenging clinical problem as patients are often exposed to several toxins and may suffer thermal injury to the respiratory tract as well. A number of chronic respiratory conditions have been described following acute inhalation injuries. Chronic airflow obstruction has been reported in patients exposed to ammonia chloride, nitrogen oxide, and sulphur dioxide. Bronchiolitis obliterans may follow exposure to nitrogen dioxide and sulphur dioxides [4].

Animal studies [12, 13] dealing with alveolar macrophage dysfunction and inhalation injury demonstrate reduced basal secretion of TNF-α, pointing to a functional down-regulation of phagocytosis.

Diagnosis

Early indication of inhalation injury is most often observed in patients referred to a burns unit and treated with mechanical ventilation at the primary hospital. The combination of clinical and laboratory findings combined with computer-derived respiratory parameters and daily bronchoscopic examination in most cases establishes the diagnosis within a few hours after the trauma. In a study of 523 residential fire fatalities in Maryland over a 6-year period, 85% of victims had blood alcohol levels greater than 0.1% and 60% carboxyhemoglobin levels greater than 60% [15]. Indication of unconsciousness with elevated carbon monoxide levels is significant when evaluating the prognosis of a burns case.

Although mucosal sloughing may be present shortly after the incident, physiological alterations will not occur until oedema is sufficient to produce airway obstruction several hours later. Consequently, fibreoptic bronchoscopy and laryngoscopy need to be repeated serially during the first 48 h when positive findings apart from oedema are inflammation, mucosal necrosis, the presence of soot and charring in the airway. To identify areas of airway trapping caused by small airway obstruction, Xenon 133 scanning is used and areas of decreased washout from alveoli demonstrated. The scan should be performed before the fourth postburn day as clearance returns to normal within this period [16].

Inhalation injuries in burn cases require clinical assessment, bronchoscopy and blood gas control whereas admission chest radiographs are insensitive indicators of airway and parenchymal lung damage [17].

Treatment strategies

Despite advances in mechanical ventilatory support, including the use of high frequency flow-interruption ventilators, inhalation injury alone [7] may increase mortality by as much as 20%, and 60% when pneumonia develops. Ventilation abnormalities are elicited primarily by large and small airway epithelial lesions whereas alveolar damage resulting in oxygenation abnormalities is more seldom. In severe cases with toxic pulmonary oedema (nitric acid), a combination of extracorporeal membrane oxygenation, use of surfactant and low dose inhalation therapy, including nitric oxide, is indicated even though outcome is poor.

When high ventilation pressures are necessary the condition may be complicated with barotrauma and necrotizing tracheobronchitis, leading to oxygenation difficulties after a few weeks' ventilation treatment. Early identification of such patients allows referral to centralized treatment units with the possibility of advanced oxygenation therapy. High frequency percussive ventilation (HFPV) improves pulmonary function and gas exchange [18, 19].

Pretreatment with aminophylline has been shown to protect against various types of acute lung injury. Mechanisms responsible are multifactorial but are thought to involve upregulation of cAMP [20] where direct antipermeability effects of cAMP on cellular contraction may protect against phosgene-induced lung injury. Early treatment with aerosolized specific antibodies may prove valuable in humans against toxin-elicited airway epithelial necrosis whereas corticosteroids have not been proven to protect the lung from the acute physiological consequences of inhalation injury [21].

A combination of aerosolized heparin and a mucolytic agent, acetyl-cysteine, prevents cellular cast formations in upper airways, thus reducing secondary pulmonary failure and mortality (heparin, 5 000 IU+20% acetyl cysteine every 4 h for 1 week) [22]. Infusion of an iron chelator (deferoxamine) in starch administered after serious smoke exposure in adult sheep significantly attenuates airway damage and systemic inflammatory injury, indicating free iron release and subsequent increase in oxidant activity [23].

Data substantiate that patients suffering from inhalation injury have higher fluid and sodium requirements than patients with external burns alone and that an increased body surface area must be entered into the Parkland formula for these cases (5.76 vs. 3.98 ml/kg/% TBA and 0.94 vs. 0.68 mEq/kg/% TBA [24]).

Long-term consequences

The improvement in survival [18] of patients with inhalation injury represents the aggregate effects of the general improvement and outcome of all burned patients, the prevention of pneumonia by high-frequency ventilation, and the reduced mortality from the pneumonias that occur. One recent Canadian paper [25] focusing upon burn survivors with inhalation injuries diagnosed with bronchscopy (n=23) concludes that pulmonary function and bronchial responsiveness (provocative concentrations of histamine resulting in a 20% fall in FEV1) were within normal ranges, as were other respiratory and cardiac variables in these patients, indicating that, in burn patients, smoke inhalation from a single domestic fire does not necessarily imply long-term respiratory health consequences.

Prevention measures

During a 10-year period in Scotland [26] 168 child deaths occurred in 118 house fires; 40% of the fires involved the 0 to 5-year age group and started as a direct result of the action of the children. The careless disposal of smoking materials was the most frequent cause and upholstery and bedding the first ignition material, leading to death as a result of smoke inhalation. The authors emphasize the importance of "self escape" which, in this age group, requires the assistance of adults and supervision and provision of a safe environment, especially in a particular socioeconomic context. Furthermore, the introduction of water sprinkler systems and low price early smoke detectors may reduce mortality in house fires.

The World Trade Center bombing disaster [11] underlines the importance of the following safety systems during high-rise building fires:
- smoke control systems with separate emergency power sources;
- lift-car position monitoring system;
- lift-car communication system with separate emergency power sources;

- two-way emergency communication system on each floor;
- stairwells with emergency lighting designed for rapid egress of crowds;
- evacuation systems/equipment to assist evacuation;
- regularly scheduled safety training and evacuation drills.

Fatal accidents originating from in-flight cabin fires comprise about 1% of all fatal accidents in the civil jet transport fleet. Nevertheless, the impossibility of escape during flight accentuates the hazards resulting from low visibility and toxic gases. Control of combustion products in an aircraft cabin is affected by several characteristics that make this environment unique [27]. The aircaraft fuselage is pressurized in flight and has an air distribution system which provides ventilation jets from the ceiling level air inlets running along the cabin length. Experimental results indicate that buoyancy effects cause smoke movement behaviour that is not predicted by traditional design analyses and flight test methodologies. Augmenting available ventilation for smoke control remains a design and safety challenge.

References

1. Crawford ME, Rask H (1996) Prehospital care of the burned patient. Eur J Emerg Med 3:247-251
2. American Burns Association (1990) Hospital and prehospital resources for optimal care of patients with burn injury: guidelines for development of and operation of burn centers. J Burn Care Rehabil 11:98-104
3. Bizovi KE, Leikin JD (1995) Smoke inhalation among firefighters. Occup Med 10(4):721-733
4. Ruddy RM (1994) Smoke inhalation injury. Pediatr Clin North Am 41(2):317-336
5. Weiss SM, Lakshminarayan S (1994) Acute inhalation injury. Clin Chest Med 15(1):103-116
6. Bucek S, Echun DA (1994) Inhalation injury by paraffin flames. Acta Chir Plast 36(3):74-76
7. Jones J, McMullen MJ, Dougherty J (1987) Toxic smoke inhalation: cyanide poisoning in fire victims. Am J Emerg Med 5(4):317-321
8. Kinsella J (1988) Smoke inhalation. Burns 14(4):269-279
9. Leveque B, Lareng L, Julien H, Lavaud J, Wassermann D, Latarjet J (1993) Child victims of house fires in France. Mortality, morbidity, prevention. Bull Acad Natl Med 177(7):1233-1239
10. Fitzpatrick JC, Cioffi WG, Cheu HW, Pruitt BA (1994) Predicting ventilation failure in children with inhalation injury. J Pediatr Surg 29(8):1122-1126
11. Quenemoen LE, Davis YM, Malilay J, Sinks T, Noji EK, Klitzman S (1996) The World Trade Center bombing: injury prevention strategies for high-rise building fires. Disasters 20(2):125-132
12. Lalonde C, Demling R, Brain J, Blanchard J (1994) Smoke inhalation injury in sheep is caused by the particle phase, not the gas phase. J Appl Physiol 77(1):15-22
13. Bidani A, Wang CZ, Heming TA (1996) Early effects of smoke inhalation on alveolar macrophage functions. Burns 22(2):101-106
14. Ghio AJ, Kennedy TP, Hatch GE, Tepper JS (1991) Reduction of neutrophil influx diminishes lung injury and mortality following phosgene inhalation. J Appl Physiol 71(2):657-665

15. Birky MM, Clarke FB (1981) Inhalation of toxic products from fires. Bull NY Acad Med 57:997-1013
16. Herndon DN, Langner F, Thompson P, Liares HA, Stein M, Traber DL (1987) Pulmonary injury in burned patients. Surg Clin North Am 67(1):31-46
17. Wittram C, Kenny JB (1994) The admission chest radiograph after acute inhalation injury and burns. Br J Radiol 67(800):751-754
18. Rue LW, Cioffi WG, Mason AD, McManus WF, Pruitt BA (1993) Improved survival of burned patients with inhalation injury. Arch Surg 128(7):772-778
19. Reper P, Dankaert R, van Hille F, van Laeke P, Duinslaeger L, Vanderkelen A (1998) The usefulness of combined high-frequency percussive ventilation during acute respiratory failure after smoke inhalation. Burns 24(1):34-38
20. Niehaus GD, Kimura R, Traber LD, Herndon DN, Flynn JT (1990) Administration of a synthetic antiprotease reduces smoke-induced lung injury. J Appl Physiol 69(2):694-699
21. Nieman GF, Clark WR, Hakim T (1991) Methylprednisolone does not protect the lung from inhalation injury. Burns 17(5):384-390
22. Desai MH, Mlcak R, Richardson J, Nichols R, Herndon DN (1998) Reduction in mortality in pediatric patients with inhalation injury with aerosolized heparin/acetylcysteine therapy. J Burn Care Rehabil 19(3):210-212
23. Demling R, Lalonde C, Ikegami K (1996) Fluid resuscitation with deferoxamine hetastarch complex attenuates the lung and systemic response to smoke inhalation. Surgery 119(3):340-348
24. Navar PD, Saffle JR, Warden GD (1985) Effect of inhalation injury on fluid resuscitation requirements after thermal injury. Am J Surg 150:716-720
25. Bourbeau J, Lacasse Y, Rouleau MY, Boucher S (1996) Combined smoke inhalation and body surface burns injury does not necessarily imply long-term respiratory health consequences. Eur Resp J 9(7):1470-1474
26. Squires T, Busuttil A (1996) Can child fatalities in house fires be prevented? Inj Prev 2:109-113
27. Eklund TI (1996) In-flight cabin smoke control. Toxicology 115(1-3):135-144
28. Barillo DJ, Goode R (1996) Fire fatality study: demographics of fire victims. Burns 22(2):85-88
29. Sciuto AM, Strickland PT, Kennedy TP, Gurtner GH (1997) Postexposure treatment with aminophylline protects against phosgene-induced acute lung injury. Exp Lung Res 23(4):317-332

Chapter 13

Vasopressors and inotropes in trauma: when, where, how long

G. Berlot, G. Trillò, A. Gullo

In severely injured patients, cardiovascular function and oxygen delivery (DO_2) to the tissues can be compromised by a host of factors, including hemorrhage, multifactorial decrease of cardiac output (CO), increased total peripheral vascular resistances (PVR), tension pneumothorax, and cardiac trauma. Thus, hypovolemia, albeit impotant, is not the only cause of reduced tissue blood flow, consequently, maintenance of blood volume may be considered part of a more complex therapeutic approach aimed at restoring tissue oxygenation, which may include the use of inotropes and/or vasoactive drugs. Many investigations have been focused on the importance of a correct triage of trauma patients, prompt identification of sources of bleeding, choice of resuscitation fluids and the role of early reparative surgery in order to maximally reduce or totally avoid the low-flow time. However, less attention has been devoted to the role of vasoactive drugs in re-establishing normoxia in trauma victims. This is in sharp contrast to other fields of critical care medicine (i.e., sepsis, cardiac failure), in which inotropes and vasoactive drugs are considered first-line agents.

Indications for treatment

For a long time hemorrhage was recognized as the basic pathophysiologic mechanism underlying trauma-induced tissue hypoxia, and thus the easily appreciated signs and symptoms of anemia and hypovolemia were considered as reliable therapeutic indicators. However, more recent investigations demonstrated that, in critically ill patients affected by different disorders, tissue dysoxia can persist and become further aggravated despite normalization of the commonly measured hemodynamic and metabolic variables [1]. Thus, it appears that the time-honored signs of shock, such as arterial hypotension, tachypnea, and tachycardia, represent the tip of an iceberg which is much deeper than previously appreciated [2]. Although many diagnostic techniques have been developed for the early detection of tissue hypoxia, for some of them widespread use at the bedside (or at the scene of the trauma) is not to be expected [3]. Actually, moving from the macrovascular down to the microvascular level, the more in-depth the search for the causes of disturbances in tissue oxygenation, the more likely it is that they will be found. It is then possible to list, in order of increasing sensitivity and specificity, the conventional and advanced parameters that must be evaluated (Table 1). However, it must

Table 1. Levels of investigation

Conventional variables
- Arterial pressure
- Central venous pressure
- Heart rate
- Urine output
- Mental status
- Skin temperature
- Hemoglobin/hematocrit

Macrocirculatory variables
- Cardiac output
- SVO_2, DO_2, VO_2, O_2er

Microcirculatory variables
- Base deficit, anion gap
- Blood lactate value
- Veno/arterial CO_2 gradient
- Gastric intramucosal CO_2/pH

be clear that new developments do not totally replace the older monitoring tools and that it is important to recognize the indication and limitations of each measured variable [4].

As far as heart rate (HR), mean arterial pressure (MAP), central venous pressure (CVP), and pulmonary artery occlusive pressure (PAOP) are concerned, it is worthwhile noting that: a) these parameters are influenced by factors other than hypovolemia or tissue dysoxia, including pain, anxiety, preexisting pulmonary or cardiovascular dysfunction and the use of cardiovascular medications; and b) their changes can occur later, when the most vulnerable tissues (i.e., the intestinal mucosa) are already dysoxic [5]. The same considerations apply for skin apperance, urinary output and mental status; in trauma patients this latter variable can be particularly unreliable due to the frequently concomitant presence of head injuries or intoxication. A more-in-depth level of investigation can provide more valuable information, yet still reflect macrocirculatory events. Several investigations addressed the effects of manipulations of DO_2 and oxygen consumption (VO_2) in trauma patients. In general, patients who survived or did not develop multiple organ dysfunction syndrome (MODS) had higher-than-normal DO_2 and VO_2 values [1, 6-8], despite similar or even less severe injuries than those assessed using the currently used severity scores. Interestingly, the time frame of resuscitation appeared to play a major role, as in survivors these values were obtained within 24 h of admission. On the basis of these findings, supranormal DO_2 and VO_2 values have been indicated as valuable therapeutic indicators in evaluating trauma as well as other categories of critically ill patients. This approach has more recently been questioned by other authors [9], who challenged the hypothesis that elevated DO_2 (>600 ml/min/m^2) and VO_2 (>150 ml/min/m^2) values in trauma patients were associated with a better outcome, as compared to patients resuscitated by conventional means. These authors failed to observe any increased survival and/or reduction of organ failure in the treatment group, reflecting what has been demonstrated in other critically ill patients, that the stress imposed upon the cardiovascular system to reach supranormal oxygen variables resulted in no benefit or was even detrimental [10]. Thus, it appears that an invasive cardiovascular monitoring is indicated, and sometimes mandatory, not to administer fluids and drugs to achieve sopranormal values, but rather to monitor the time course and evolution of the cardiovascular response and to promptly identify and correct any derangement. This could be particularly important: a) in elderly patients and in subjects with limited cardiovascular or renal reserve, in whom an overzealous fluid resuscitation can be detrimental, and b) in younger patients with severe blood loss [11].

Other goals of treatment include variables associated with the oxygenation status of the tissues. Serial blood lactate determinations are valuable in trauma patients, as not only the peak values but also their time decay have been associated with a better outcome and a reduced incidence of organ failure, underscoring again the importance of the initial resuscitation [12]. However, other studies failed to correlate blood lactate levels with changes of the anion gap (AG) and/or base excess (BE), indicating that anions other than lactate are involved in the pathogenesis of trauma-associated metabolic acidosis and that BE and AG should both be considered if the redox status is used to titrate the resuscitation [13]. At a more-indepth level, the enteric mucosa is particularly vulnerable to hypoxia as compared to other tissues [5] and it has been experimentally demonstrated that hemorrhagic shock is associated with decreased gastric mucosal pH (pHi) [14]. Thus, several investigations were aimed at monitoring this variable and the effects of its manipulation. Even if the overall results indicated that in trauma patients and in other categories of critically ill patients this variable can be abnormal, even in the absence of other signs of tissue dysoxia [15], the effect of pHi-oriented therapy in the resucitation of trauma remains controversial [15, 16].

The role of cardiovascular drugs

It is clear that in trauma patients the first resuscitative efforts should be directed toward arresting the bleeding and re-establishing an appropriate hemoglobin level [17]. The role of inotropes is less clear, at least in the absence of precise indications of their use, as can occur in elderly patients with a limited cardiac or renal reserve, in whom an approach entirely based on the fluid administration is not safely feasible. It is therefore worthwhile to identify a subset of patients who could benefit from inotropes even in the absence of these limitations and to choose a drug with a more favorable risk-benefit ratio. Unfortunately, the results coming from clinical investigations can be confounding, as the studies vary in terms of patients enrolled, end points of treatment and drug(s) used. In severely head injured patients with multiple trauma, Scalea et al. [18] observed that, when the CO failed to increase in response to fluids, the use of inotropes with vasodilating properties (dobutamine), with or without dopamine, was followed by the correction of the considered cardiovascular parameters without any concomitant increase in intracranial pressure (ICP). Also, Abou-Khalil et al. [11] advocated the early use of inotropes, targeted at invasively measured hemodynamic variables, in young trauma patients, claiming that a hidden trauma-induced myocardial depression, not reflected by CVP, MAP and HR, can persist for a long time in the post-acute phase. However, these conclusions can be considered somewhat controversial, as other investigations led to different conclusions, not indicating the extensive use of inotropes. Miller et al. [19] prospectively studied trauma patients with a reduced right ventricular ejection fraction who were treated with inotropes or with volume loading targeted to increase their preload, which was assessed by the changes in the right ventricular end-diastolic volume (RVEDV). Gut perfusion was evaluated by means of the pHi. Despite similar increases in oxygen variables, rate of complications and days on ventilator, fluid-resuscitated patients had significantly better splanchnic perfusion, without any of the expected pulmonary complications. The importance of preload is further underlined by Chang et al. [15], who observed that supranormal levels of RVEDV were associated with a better outcome in injured patients.

Another crucial point is the choice of the inotrope. As the administration of inotropes with vasodilating properties might not be free of risk in hypovolemic patients, it appears that a combination of drugs with vasodilating and vasoconstricting properties could be beneficial in these circumstances. A dopamine-dobutamine combination could be particularly useful, as it allows maintenance of MAP without any significant increase in PAOP [20]. As far as the splanchnic circulation is concerned, the effects of inotropes are less clear, as, once again, the results of both experimental and clinical investigations led to different results, showing that the same drug can exert different effects in different categories of patients. As an example, whereas Silverman et al. [21] observed an increase in pHi in septic patients given dobutamine, other investigators, studying a group of postoperative cardiac surgery patients, failed to observe any change and attributed this effect to a dissociation between total splanchinc blood flow and that directed to the mucosa [22, 23]. Despite these shortcomings, persistent reduction of pHi has been associated with a worse outcome in critically ill patients, including those admitted with severe trauma [24-27]. However, despite these results, the precise role of pHi, used as a monitoring tool and as a variable to titrate therapy, has not been established yet in trauma patients. Due to its elevated cost, it is likely that the major role for measuring pHi might be reserved for the post-acute phase [28], when splanchinc hypoxia might not be reflected by the currently measured hemodynamic parameters [29]. In earlier phases, especially in shocked patients, the same information about visceral hypoxemia can be easily infererred, at an extremely lower cost, by blood gas analysis [30].

The role of vasopressors in the treatment of trauma patients is limited to the restoration and maintenance of the perfusion pressure in some vital regions. As it has been demonstrated that both hypoxia and arterial hypotension occur frequently in head trauma patients, with hypotension being more difficult to treat [31], the use of vasopressors has been advocated to prevent the reduction of cerebral perfusion associated either with a trauma-related increase of the ICP [32] or that associated with the initiation of mechanical ventilation [33]. Other indications as to the use of pressors include arterial hypotension unresponsive to volume resuscitation and inotropes.

Conclusions

From the current evidence, it appears that the use of inotropes in trauma patients is indicated in two circumstances:
1. in the early phase of treatment, when fluid resuscitation alone is not able to restore normoxia, as indicated by the currently used diagnostic tools. In this phase, the use, albeit temporary, of vasopressors should be considered;
2. in a more advanced phase, when there is biochemical and/or instrumental evidence of tissue dysoxia, even in the absence of macrocirculatory derangement.
In both cases, appropriate monitoring of the effect of the medications is mandatory.

References

1. Moore FA, Haenel JB, Moore EE, Whitehill TA (1992) Incommensurate oxygen consumption in response to maximal oxygen availability predicts postinjury multiple organ failure. J Trauma 33:58-67
2. Gutierrez G, Bismar H, Dantzker DR, Silva N (1992) Comparison of gastric intramucosal pH with oxygen transport and consumption in criticall ill patients. Crit Care Med 20: 451-457
3. Hess D, Kacmarek RM (1993) Techniques and devices for monitoring oxygenation. Resp Care 38:646-671
4. Cornwell EE, Kennedy F, Rodriguez J (1996) The critical care of the severely injured patient: assessing and improving oxygen delivery. Surg Clin North Am 76:959-969
5. Fink MP (1991) Gastrointestinal mucosal injury in experimental models of shock, trauma and sepsis. Crit Care Med 19:627-641
6. Bishop MH, Shoemaker WC, Appel PL et al (1995) Prospective randomized trial of survivor values of cardiac index, oxygen delivery and oxygen consumption as resuscitation endpoints in severe trauma. J Trauma 38:780-785
7. Shoemaker WC, Appel P, Kram H et al (1988) Prospective trial of supranormal values of survivors as therapeutic goals in high risk surgical patients. Chest 94:1176-1186
8. Shoemaker WC, Appel P, Kram H et al (1990) The efficacy of central venous and pulmonary artery catheters and therapy based upon them in reducing mortality and morbidity. Arch Surg 125:1332-1338
9. Durham RM, Neunaber K, Mazusky J, Shapiro MJ, Baue AE (1996) The use of oxygen consumption and delivery as endpoints for resuscitation in critically ill patients. J Trauma 41:32-40
10. Hayes MA, Timmins AC, Yau EHS et al (1994) Elevation of systemic oxygen delivery in the treatmetn of criticall ill patients. New Engl J Med 330:1717-1722
11. Abou-Khalil B, Scalea TM, Trookin SZ, Henry SM, Hitchcock R (1994) Hemodynamic responses to shock in young trauma patients: need for invasive monitoring. Crit Care Med 22:633-639

12. Manikis P, Jankowsky S, Zhang H, Khan RJ, Vincent LJ (1995) Correlation of blood lactate levels to organ failure and mortality after trauma. Am J Emerg Med 13:619-622
13. Mikulshek A, Henry SM, Donovan R, Scalea TM (1996) Serum lactate is not predicted by anion gap or base excess after trauma resuscitation. J Trauma 40:218-224
14. Yee JB, McJames SW (1994) Use of gastric intramucosal pH as a monitor during hemorrhagic shock. Circ Shock 43:44-48
15. Chang MC, Cheatham ML, Nelson LD, Rutherford EJ, Morris JA (1994) Gastric tonometry supplements information provided by systemic indicators of oxygen transport. J Trauma 37:488-494
16. Ruomen RMH, Vreugde JPC, Goris JA (1994) Gastric tonometry in multiple trauma patients. J Trauma 36:313-316
17. Trunkey DD (1991) Initial treatment of patients with severe trauma. New Engl J Med 324:1259-1263
18. Scalea TM, Maltz S, Jelon J, Trooskin SZ, Duncan AO, Sclafani SJA (1994) Resuscitation of multiple trauma and head injury: role of crystalloid fluids and inotropes. Crit Care Med 22:1610-1615
19. Miller PR, Meredith JW, Chang MC (1998) Randomized, prospective comparison of incresed preload versus inotrpes in the resuscitation of trauma patients: effects on cardiopulmonary function and visceral perfusion. J Trauma 44:107-113
20. Domsky MF, Wilson RF (1993) hemodynamic resuscitation. Crit Care Clin 10:715-726
21. Silverman HJ, Tuma P (1992) Gastric tonometry in patients with sepsis: effects of dobutamine infusions and packed red blood cell transfusions. Chest 102:184-188
22. Parviainen I, Ruokonen E, Takala J (1995) Dobutamine-induced dissociation between changes in splanchnic blood flow and gastric intramucosal pH after cardiac surgery. Br J Anaesth 74:277-282
23. Uusaro A, Ruokonen E, Takala J (1995) Gastric intramucosal pH does not reflect changes in splanchnic blood flow after cardiac surgery. Br J Anaesth 74:149-154
24. Mythen MG, Webb AR (1994) Intra-operative gut mucosal hypoperfusion is associated with increased post-operative complications and costs. Intensive Care Med 20:99-104
25. Doglio G, Pusajo J, Egurrola M et al (1991) Gastric mucosal pH as a prognostic index of mortality in critically ill patients. Crit Care Med 19:1037-1040
26. Marik PE (1993) Gastric intramucosal pH: a better predictor of multiorgan dysfuntion syndrome and death than oxygen derived variables in patients with sepsis. Chest 104:225-229
27. Gutierrez G, Palizas F, Doglio G et al (1992) Gastric intramucosal pH as a therapeutic index of tissue oxygenation in critically ill patients. Lancet 339:195-199
28. Ivatury RR, Simon RJ, Havriliak D, Garcia C, Greenbarg J, Stahl WM (1995) Gastric mucosal pH and oxygen delivery and oxygen consumption indices in the assessment of adequacy of resuscitation after trauma: a prosepctive randomized study. J Trauma 39:128-136
29. Maynard N, Bihari D, Beale R, Smithies M, Baldock G, Mason R, McColl I (1993) Assessment of splanchnic oxygenation by gastric tonometry in patients with acute circulatory failure. JAMA 270:1203-1210
30. Boyd O, Mackay CJ, Lamb G, Bland JM, Grounds RM, Bennett ED (1993) Comparison of clinical information gained from routine blood-gas analysis and from gastric tonometry for intramural pH. Lancet 341:142-146
31. Stocchetti N, Furlan A, Volta A (1996) Hypoxemia and arterial hypotension at the accident scene in head injury. J Trauma 40:764-767

32. Stocchetti N, Paparella A, Serioli T, Giulioni M, Vezzani A (1992) Increasing the pressure of cerebral perfusion to control intracranial pressure. Minerva Anestesiol 58(Suppl 1): 165-171
33. Franklin C, Samuel J, Hu TC (1994) Life-threatening hypotension associated with emergency intubation and initiation of mechanical ventilation. Am J Emerg Med 12:425-428

Chapter 14

Creating a trauma anaesthesia service

M.J.A. PARR, J.P. NOLAN, G. DESJARDINS

Trauma anaesthesia refers to a speciality within anaesthesia that exists to manage the victims of trauma. As such it should be differentiated from anaesthesia for trauma. The emphasis is on preservation of life and limb through resuscitation, the provision of analgesia, surgical anaesthesia and critical care. Trauma anaesthesia has special requirements in terms of facility and personnel, and encompasses management of the trauma patient from the time of injury until discharge from a critical care facility.

A Trauma Anaesthesia Service may arise within an existing emergency anaesthesia service or may be developed as a separate service. In either case it must be recognised that to be effective a Trauma Anaesthesia Service must be an integral component of a trauma system.

Facility requirements

Avoidable morbidity and mortality from major trauma has been repeatedly recognised to arise from a number of causes which include: inadequate pre-hospital care, inappropriate in-hospital resuscitation, delayed surgery and inappropriate management by individuals with inadequate experience [1-3]. Trauma centres and systems have been developed as a long term, cost effective method of delivering state of the art trauma care to reduce avoidable morbidity and mortality. Trauma systems provide identified levels of care, maximise the utilisation of existing resources, concentrate clinical skills and integrate the pre-hospital, hospital, and rehabilitative phases of trauma care.

The trauma centre should provide a facility in which trauma anaesthesia can be performed to a level of excellence. In the majority of settings there should be helicopter as well as land ambulance access. The facility should have easy transfer to an admitting/resuscitation area with a wide range of equipment necessary for the provision of safe anaesthesia, ventilation and circulatory resuscitation of trauma patients. The staff necessary for a trauma team response should be immediately available (see below). Operating rooms and radiology imaging facilities should be situated adjacent to the admitting area. A post-anaesthesia recovery area and critical care facility should also be close by. Offices, administrative assistance, a clinical computer system and the other services necessary to support a Trauma Anaesthesia Service will also be required.

A level 1 trauma centre as defined by the American College of Surgeons and the

Joint Commission on Accreditation of Healthcare Organisations is the sort of facility that will require and be able to support the concept of a Trauma Anaesthesia Service [4] (Table 1).

Table 1. Facility characteristics for a level 1 Trauma Anaesthesia Service

- Commitment to excellent care of trauma patients
- Reliable communication systems
- Sufficient case load (>600 cases per year)
- At least 50 severely injured patients for each specialist anaesthetist per year
- 24 h immediate availability of staff experienced in trauma care (anaesthetists, anaesthetic assistants, emergency physicians, surgeons (general, orthopaedic, neuro, nurses, operating room staff)
- 24 h availability of a resuscitation area
- 24 h availability of an operating room available for trauma
- 24 h radiology service (including CT and angiography)
- 24 h blood bank and laboratory support
- 24 h recovery and critical care facility
- Quality assurance, audit and risk management
- Teaching and training programmes
- Trauma research programme
- Public education and trauma prevention

Personnel requirements

Anaesthetists are unique in that they can provide continuity of care for the severely injured patient from the pre-hospital phase, through the emergency department/resuscitation area, the operating room and into critical care. It is rare however that this potential is realised in practice.

The roles undertaken by anaesthesiologists managing trauma patients vary between institutions and different countries. The roles of the trauma anaesthetist are summarised in Table 2. As a defined service in the trauma system it should be possible to identify individuals and their specific roles within the Trauma Anaesthesia Service (Table 3).

Trauma Anaesthesia Services should provide 24 h cover by anaesthetists specifically trained in the management of trauma patients. This requirement may be fulfilled by non-resident specialist staff provided they can be in the hospital at the time of the patients arrival, or shortly after. Experienced trainee staff should be available in house 24 h a day and, ideally, specialist trauma anaesthetists should also be resident when on call. This is important because the skills of a specialist trauma anaesthetist will often be required immediately upon admission. Up to 20% of major trauma patients may require intubation within 1 h of admission, many of them as an emergency because of airway compromise with potential cervical spine injury and with associated cardiovascular instability. Around 10% of major trauma patients will require emergency surgery. The skills and experience of a specialist

Table 2. Roles of the trauma anaesthetist

- Pre-hospital care
- In-hospital trauma patient resuscitation as a member of the trauma team
- Trauma team leader
- The provision of analgesia (acute pain service)
- Anaesthesia in the operating room
- Pre and post-operative critical care
- Physician for the transfer of a trauma patient
- Training and education
- Research and audit
- Trauma prevention
- Disaster planning

Table 3. Personnel within a Trauma Anaesthesia Service

- A clinical director of Trauma Anaesthesia
- Specialists with responsibility for clinical service, equipment, education, training, research, audit and quality assurance
- Fellowship appointers
- Trainers in Trauma Anaesthesia
- Certified Registered Nurse Anaesthetist (USA)
- Trained anaesthetic assistants
- Administrative and support staff

trauma anaesthetist are particularly important during this crucial period. To attain these skills the trauma anaesthetist will require a period of specialist training in an appropriate facility (see below).

The individual skills of the trauma anaesthetist are common to all fields of anaesthetic practice. However, because of the urgency of the situation, the lack of time for full assessment and deliberation, and the complexity of the cases, trauma anaesthetists will find themselves utilising these skills more frequently than other anaesthetic sub-specialists (Table 4).

Table 4. Individual skills of the trauma anaesthetist

- Ability to rapidly establish priorities
- Ability to treat and diagnose simultaneously
- Ability to work in adverse circumstances with patients that are often severely compromised
- Ability to lead or work as part of a team
- Experience in difficult airway, ventilation and circulatory support
- Experience in a wide range of anaesthesia skills
- Experience in a wide range of analgesia techniques
- Familiarity with a wide range of critical care procedures
- Ability to deal with a high number of critical incidents

Although the workload of the trauma anaesthetist can be very variable, it is common to have periods of high physical and psychological stress. In the past, trauma anaesthesia has been labelled as a low status subspecialty and has received little support from the anaesthesia profession. Anaesthetists have often preferred not to treat trauma patients. Factors influencing this have included: the impact of trauma call coverage on their private lives, a greater time commitment required for care, low financial compensation, a perceived increased liability risk, and an adverse impact on private practice. To an extent, this is changing and the development of the trauma anaesthesia specialist with a professional, credible status may be part of the reason for this. Unfortunately, as yet, the American Society of Anesthesiologists does not recognise Trauma Anaesthesia as a subspecialty.

Pre-hospital care

An effective trauma system begins in the pre-hospital setting. The ultimate survival of a significant number of patients depends on their pre-hospital management. The pre-hospital emergency medical service (EMS) system needs short response times, adequately trained individuals with the right equipment, and the full support of communications and hospital facilities. The trauma anaesthetist has roles in the training of pre-hospital EMS personnel and, in some countries, may be part of the pre-hospital response.

There are controversies in pre-hospital trauma management concerning the type of pre hospital provider and the interventions they perform. Like the EMS in the United States (US), the United Kingdom (UK) and Australia utilise a paramedic based system. In the UK, ambulance technicians are trained in basic airway management, cervical spine control, and shock advisory defibrillation. Paramedics have the additional skills of tracheal intubation, intravenous cannulation, fluid therapy and use of intravenous analgesia [5]. In other parts of Europe (France, Germany, and Belgium) ambulance technicians are supported by physicians, usually anaesthesiologists, in mobile intensive care units. Supplemental skills provided by physicians in general, and anaesthesiologists in particular, include the use of neuromuscular blocking drugs and a broad range of analgesics and fluids, insertion of chest drains, cricothyroidotomy, and the ability to triage the patient to the most appropriate hospital. In theory, the doctor's ability to provide a more sophisticated and individualised continuum of patient care (not necessarily protocol driven) in the initial hospital phase may expedite definitive care. Certainly the French anaesthesiologists working within the Service D'Aide Medicale Urgente (SAMU) strongly support this hypothesis [6]. Unfortunately, there are no good randomised controlled trials proving that the outcome for trauma patients is influenced by the type of pre-hospital provider or even the procedures performed. There are only small, retrospective, observational studies which have produced conflicting results [7-12]. Some studies have suggested that Advanced Life Support (ALS) procedures improve physiological variables but not outcome [13]. One of the problems with pre-hospital trauma studies is the lack of a uniform system or set of definitions for reporting results. A working group has been convened to develop "Guidelines for

Uniform Recording and Reporting of Performance and Outcome Following Trauma" very much along the lines of the Utstein template for the reporting of pre-hospital cardiac arrest [14]. It is hoped that this will enhance the ability to compare data derived from different EMS systems.

Communication

Communication is vital in providing an efficient link between pre-hospital and in-hospital trauma patient resuscitation. The importance of having advanced warning before the arrival of a severely injured patient cannot be overstated. Ideally, the pre-hospital personnel at the scene should be able to communicate directly with the trauma team leader via a talk-through link. This provides concise and essential information on the patient's condition and the estimated time of arrival at hospital. The trauma team leader can give advice on triage and intervention if required and can then decide whether to activate the trauma team. Many hospitals will have specific criteria for a trauma team call similar to the criteria used by pre-hospital personnel to triage patients to trauma centres (Table 5). With advance warning, medical and nursing staff can prepare a resuscitation bay or operating room for the patient's arrival.

Table 5. Criteria for triage of adult trauma patients to the Ryder Trauma Centre

- Systolic BP <90 mm Hg
- Respiratory rate <10 or >29
- Glasgow Coma Score <13
- Penetrating trauma: head, neck, trunk
- Acute paralysis
- Second or third degree burns >14% total body surface area
- Traumatic amputation proximal to wrist or ankle
- Ejection from motor vehicle accident
- "Special" paramedic decision
- Trauma centre decision

Roles of the trauma anaesthetist

In-hospital trauma resuscitation

Up to 90% of major trauma patients do not initially require surgery. The trauma anaesthetist has particular skills in airway and ventilatory management and circulatory support. These make him the most appropriate clinician to be primarily involved with trauma patient resuscitation. In most countries this individual plays a vital but variable role within the trauma team (Table 6). However, a recent survey of level 1 trauma centres in the US showed that an anaesthesiologist was included routinely on the trauma team in only 30% of cases [15]. In many institutions air-

Table 6. Role of the anaesthetist in trauma patient resuscitation for different countries

	Pre-hospital EMS	Team leader	IV access	Invasive procedure[a]	Airway	Lab data[b] interpretation	Diagnosis
Australia	+	±	+	+	+	+	+
Austria	+	+	+	+	+	+	+
Chile	–	–	+	+	+	–	–
England	±	±	+	+	+	±	±
France	+	+	+	+	+	+	+
Germany	+	+	+	+	+	+	+
Italy	±	±	+	+	+	±	±
Japan	–	–	±	±	±	–	–
Mexico	–	–	–	–	–	–	–
Netherlands	±	–	±	±	±	–	–
Norway	+	–	+	+	+	±	–
Switzerland	+	–	+	+	+	±	–
USA	–	–	±	±	±	±	–

+ Anaesthetists play a major role; – Anaesthetists play a minimal role; ± Anaesthetists have a variable role; *EMS*, Emergency Medical Service; *IV*, Intravenous
[a] Invasive procedures such as inserting chest tubes, urinary catheters, arterial lines
[b] Laboratory data interpretation–leading role for anaesthetist

way management during trauma patient resuscitation is performed primarily by emergency physicians [16]. Failure to inform anaesthesia specialists that patients have entered the EMS system and the absence of an anaesthetist as a formal member of the trauma team will result in avoidable morbidity and mortality. An effective Trauma Anaesthesia Service should include the trauma anaesthetist as a key/lead member of the trauma team.

The trauma team

Trauma patient resuscitation is most efficient if undertaken by a team of appropriately trained doctors and nurses. In this way a variety of tasks can be undertaken simultaneously, a process "known as horizontal organisation". The trauma team should be alerted prior to the patients arrival to allow time for assembly and preparation. The precise composition of the team will inevitably vary from one hospital to another. The composition of a typical team and the team member's roles are listed in Table 7.

Table 7. Composition of a typical trauma team

- Team leader: primary and secondary surveys, co-ordination of team, overall responsibility for the patient while in the Emergency Department
- Anaesthetist: airway, ventilation, central venous access, difficult peripheral access, fluid balance, analgesia
- Other doctor: all other procedures, chest drain, fracture splinting, urethral catheter
- Nurses: measure vital signs, record data, remove clothes, assist doctors
- Radiographer: cervical spine, chest, and pelvic x-rays, other x-rays as requested by team leader
- Porter: to take samples to pathology labs, to retrieve urgent blood from blood bank

The trauma anaesthetist as the trauma team leader

The team leader plays a vital role in co-ordinating the activities of the rest of the trauma team. This person must be experienced in trauma patient resuscitation and must be capable of liasing with all the relevant specialists. In many European countries this role is often taken by an appropriately experienced anaesthesiologist, although this is rarely the case in the US [15]. The anaesthetist has credentials every bit as valid as the trauma surgeon or emergency physician for the job of team leader, provided he has undergone appropriate training. By taking on the role of the trauma team leader the trauma anaesthetist will increase his credibility within the team and increase his professional status. The role of the team leader has been defined comprehensively by a British Trauma Society Standards Working Party (Table 8) [17]. These standards represent close to an ideal situation and are probably achievable only by hospitals with relatively large trauma units. Nevertheless, it is possible to create a system on a lower level that brings senior, experienced clinicians into the trauma resuscitation room before, or soon after, the admission of a seriously injured patient.

Table 8. The role of the trauma team leader. (From [17])

- To offer advice to any hospital wishing to discuss or refer a patient, and to accept appropriate referrals
- To obtain a history from the ambulance staff (for direct admissions) or from the referring doctor and medical escort (for transferred patients)
- To examine the patient (performing a primary and secondary survey)
- To establish the priorities for investigation and intervention
- To co-ordinate the trauma team
- To maintain an overview, avoiding undue involvement in practical procedures, but intervening appropriately in critical situations
- To supervise the administration of fluids, blood, and blood products
- To provide analgesia
- To request and interpret investigations in conjunction with other team members
- To consult with or refer to other specialists where appropriate, indicating any perceived needs for urgent intervention
- To supervise spinal precautions
- To supervise the patient during transfer within the hospital and during imaging procdures
- To co-ordinate the assignment of the consultant responsible for continuing care
- To arrange transfer to the operating theatre, intensive care unit, or other ward area (or to another hospital when indicated), and to provide a detailed hand-over to their staff
- To review the patient subsequently to help maintain continuity
- To inform the family
- To excuse the Trauma Team members at the end of the resuscitation, and to debrief the team after difficult cases
- To make a detailed note in the patient's records and to record agreed information for audit

The provision of analgesia

The trauma anaesthetist has particular skills in the provision of pain relief and anaesthesia, both of vital importance in the early management of the severely injured patient. Analgesia (and anaesthesia) should be regarded as part of the resuscitation process for it brings with it not only pain relief and psychological improvement but also physiological improvement with cardiovascular stability, ventilatory improvement and subsequently improved organ and tissue perfusion [18]. Effective relief of severe pain in the compromised patient requires not only knowledge and experience of the wide variety of analgesic agents but also the skill to support the vital functions involved in respiration and the circulation which may be depressed by effective analgesic doses. The post operative trauma patient may benefit from more advanced analgesic techniques including regional local anaesthetic blocks, epidural analgesia or patient controlled analgesia (PCA). The provision of an acute pain service has in recent years become the domain of anaesthetists. It is quite appropriate that the trauma anaesthetist takes an active role in providing an acute pain service.

Anaesthesia in the operating room

The anaesthetic management of severe trauma patients in the operating room can be challenging, even for the very experienced anaesthesiologist. This is one area in which the requirement for an appropriately trained anaesthesiologist is undisputed. The patient requires ongoing resuscitation, correction or prevention of hypothermia and coagulopathy, and techniques to minimise post-operative morbidity. Anaesthesia will often require the presence of two anaesthetists and the provision of qualified anaesthetic assistance should be considered essential for the safe and efficient conduct of anaesthesia.

Post-anaesthesia care

Trauma patients should be recovered in a designated post anaesthesia care unit which should be adjacent to the operating room. The trauma anaesthetist must be immediately available. Staff trained in the care of patients recovering from anaesthesia must be present at all times. Recovery should be supervised by the anaesthetist and written protocols should be in place. The trauma anaesthetist will need to establish the level of post-operative monitoring required, the methods of pain relief, and a strategy for the management of intravenous fluids and respiratory care.

Pre- and post-operative critical care

In many countries anaesthesiologists have primary responsibility for the management of trauma patients in the critical care unit. This demands extensive knowledge and experience in multiple organ support which is relevant to any critically ill patient. This might include advanced modes of ventilation, inotropic therapy, and renal replacement therapy. Facets of care that are specific to the trauma patient include the management of head injuries, burns, and spinal trauma. The ability to evaluate complex problems, prioritise, and to communicate effectively with many disciplines is necessary for effective critical care of these challenging patients.

Attending physician for the transfer of a trauma patient

Severely injured patients frequently require intra-hospital or inter-hospital transport. The regionalization of trauma services necessitates an increase in the number of long distance trauma patient transfers. Irrespective of the distance the patient needs to be transported, there is the potential for complications unless attended by suitably experienced personnel with appropriate equipment. The accompanying doctor must be skilled in airway management and have thorough knowledge of the benefits and limitations of portable ventilators and monitors. There is little doubt that an experienced anaesthesiologist is ideally suited to this task. The Association of Anaesthetists of Great Britain and Ireland have recently published recommendations for the transfer of head-injured patients [19].

Monitoring

By any definition, major trauma patients are critically ill and it is entirely appropriate to provide monitoring in the Emergency Department/resuscitation area and operating room which is to the same standard as that on the Intensive Care Unit. If appropriate, arterial cannulae and central venous catheters should be inserted as soon as possible. Small, portable monitors that display ECG, invasive blood pressure, oxygen saturation, central venous pressure, end tidal carbon dioxide and temperature are widely available and should be used in all major trauma patients. A laboratory facility to provide a full blood count, coagulation studies, urea, creatinine and electrolytes, arterial blood gases, toxicology and cross matching of blood must be available 24 h. With the increasing sophistication and availability of point-of-care testing equipment, many of these investigations can now be done at the patient's bed side.

Training requirements for a trauma anaesthetist

Common errors are recognised in the management of trauma patients who suffer avoidable morbidity and mortality (Table 9). Formal training programmes in trauma anaesthesia will reduce the risks of these problems. However, there are no consistent training requirements for trauma anaesthesia. In some systems Advanced Trauma Life Support (ATLS) and a minimum number of continuous medical education (CME) hours in trauma are required but this is hardly comprehensive. In the past, military service was considered a good way of gaining trauma experience, both during conflict and because of the association with civilian centres during peace time. These days the military has come to rely on civilian centres for trauma experience. Most anaesthetists in training are inevitably exposed to trauma patients. But with training programmes of 4-6 years now being commonplace and limitations on the number of hours worked, many trainees see relatively few major trauma patients.

Those interested in pursuing a career in trauma anaesthesia should undertake a period of training within a trauma centre which is part of a trauma system should be required. While the duration of Fellowships vary, 12 months is ideal. A good trauma fellowship will provide clinical experience in the areas of trauma anaesthesia outlined above. Exposure to, and understanding of the role of trauma anaesthesia in Pre-hospital care, Emergency Medicine and Critical Care is a high priority. The Trauma Anaesthesia Fellowship should provide the competent trainee with the essential skills required by a Specialist Trauma Anaesthetist. These skills fall into three domains: 1) knowledge (cognitive skills); 2) practical abilities (psychomotor skills); 3) attitudes (affective skills).

Fellowships are now available at centres including: Bellevue Hospital Centre, New York University Medical School; the Trauma Hospital Lorenz Bohler, Vienna, Austria; the Clinic of Anaesthesiology, University of Mainz, Germany; the R Adams Cowley Trauma Center, Baltimore, USA; the Ryder Trauma Center, Miami, USA (Table 10); Sunnybrook Health Science Centre, Toronto, Canada; the University of California, San Francisco General Hospital, USA; SAMU de Paris, France; and Childrens Memorial Hospital, Chicago, USA. Other programmes and further details are available from ITACCS-Education, PO Box 4826, Baltimore MD 21211 USA (fax 410 235 8084).

Table 9. Common errors in trauma patient management

- Failure to adequately evaluate the patient
- Inappropriate delay of surgery
- Rushing or being rushed into inappropriate management
- Proceeding without adequate backup or resources
- Failures of communication
- Failure to anticipate problems and being unprepared

Table 10. The Trauma Anaesthesia and Critical Care Fellowship programme of the Ryder Trauma Centre, University of Miami, Florida

• Trauma anaesthesia (operating room duties)	3 months
• Trauma resuscitation	3 months
• Trauma critical care	3 months
• Research	3 months

The International Trauma Anaesthesia and Critical Care Society (ITACCS)

In Baltimore, Maryland in 1988 a group of enthusiasts for Trauma Anaesthesia established ITACCS. The society holds an annual symposium, numerous seminars, offers research grants and has been responsible for several publications on trauma anaesthesia and critical care, including what probably remains the definitive text on Trauma Anaesthesia [20]. Over 1 000 members from 44 countries are able to exchange and develop ideas on all aspects of trauma anaesthesia, resuscitation, and critical care. Information about the society can be obtained from ITACCS World Headquarters, PO Box 4826, Baltimore MD 21211, USA (fax +1 410 235 8084).

Education

Continuous medical education

Education is an essential component of the trauma system to maintain quality and ensure progress. Adequate time and financial resources should be identified to support continuing education. While it has been suggested that 20 CME hours per year in trauma related education should be considered the minimum, to achieve this in practice has often proved difficult. Trauma Anaesthesia Services need to see this as a priority and ensure that they produce programmes that will contribute to CME and also ensure that their staff are released from clinical duties so that they can achieve their CME goals.

Advanced trauma life support

A considerable advance in trauma patient resuscitation has been made by the dissemination of the ATLS course to many countries [21]. Unfortunately, it is very difficult to prove improved patient outcome and only one group has documented a reduction in trauma mortality after the introduction of ATLS [22, 23]. The ATLS course manual and slides are produced by the Committee on Trauma of the American College of Surgeons (ACS). By its very nature, the course is didactic and an identical core content is taught to all doctors on ATLS courses across the world. Inevitably there are some controversial areas, particularly in airway management [24], but many of theses issues have been, and are being, resolved in later editions of the manual.

ATLS provides a very useful framework on which we can base our resuscitation efforts. Although originally the course was aimed at the single-handed physician working in a rural hospital, the ATLS protocols are now adapted for a team approach. It is testament to the perceived utility of ATLS that since its introduction to the UK more than 9 000 individuals have attended a provider course and there are now 621 ATLS instructors. Anaesthesiologists make an important contribution to ATLS courses. In the UK, the current Chairman of the ATLS Committee is an anaesthesiologist and more ATLS instructors are from anaesthesia than from any other speciality (1997). More information on ATLS can be received from the ATLS office, Raven Education Department, RCS (telephone 0171 973 2102, fax 0171 973 2117, e-mail: atls@rcseng.ac.uk).

All trainee anaesthetists should be encouraged to complete an ATLS course, and it should be considered a requirement for a fellowship in trauma anaesthesia. ATLS

Instructor status should ideally be held by those individuals expected to function as a team leader or work as specialists in trauma anaesthesia. Some sort of educator training is required if the trauma anaesthetist is to function effectively as an educator. This training is provided very effectively by the ATLS Instructor course.

The comprehensive approach to trauma course

A Comprehensive Approach to Trauma (CAT) Course is being developed by ITACCS. It is designed to build on the basic skills and knowledge gained from ATLS. The course is aimed at the in depth early management of trauma as practised by anaesthetists, emergency physicians and critical care physicians. The CAT course will build on the success of ITACCS seminars on trauma anaesthesia and provide an accessible means for practising physicians to draw on the experience and skills of those trauma anaesthetists who deal with trauma on a daily basis. It is hoped that the course will be ready for dissemination in 1999.

Video as an educational tool

The video-recording of trauma resuscitation is used as an educational tool in many centres. In Baltimore a trauma anaesthesia teaching programme based on task analysis through video recordings interfaced with patient vital signs has been in operation for many years [25]. Through this and other work, protocols can be developed to facilitate management of trauma patients. Protocols need to be comprehensive but they should be approached with flexibility and common sense. With the increasing availability of high fidelity simulation tools, simulators and computer generated virtual reality will become increasing important to education.

Audit and research

Anyone who has ever done a Medline search on trauma anaesthesia will know of the relative lack of information on the subject in the medical literature. What information there is requires extensive searching, reflecting the lack of recognition of trauma anaesthesia as associated keywords.

Science progresses by demonstrating and eliminating errors. An effective Trauma Anaesthesia Service should contribute to this progress and will need a comprehensive audit facility to achieve this. In 1988, the Royal College of Surgeons Working Party Report on the Management of Patients with Major Injuries [1] highlighted serious deficiencies in the way trauma patients were managed in the UK [2]. At the end of the same year, in an attempt to improve evaluation of UK trauma services, a number of hospitals started to contribute data to the Major Trauma Outcome Study (MTOS; UK) [26]. This audit system had been established in the US in 1982 [27]. The first report from MTOS (UK), published in 1992, was based on 2 years of data from 33 hospitals [28]. Unfortunately, its conclusions echoed those of the Royal College of Surgeons' report 4 years earlier: "the initial management of major trauma in the United Kingdom remained unsatisfactory".

Specifically, the mortality for 6111 patients sustaining blunt trauma and treated in the 14 busiest hospitals was significantly higher than that predicted from a comparable US dataset (actual 408 vs predicted 295.6, $p<0.001$). Other key findings from this report were that 21% of patients with an Injury Severity Score (ISS) greater than 15 took longer than 1 h to reach hospital and that a junior trainee was in charge of initial hospital resuscitation in 57% of seriously injured patients.

The MTOS (UK) has now been collecting data on seriously injured patients for 8 years. There are 86 000 patients on the database and 117 hospitals in the UK have enrolled with MTOS [29]. Last year MTOS (UK) changed its name to the UK Trauma Audit and Research Network and formed links with the Cochrane Centre and the NHS Centre for Reviews and Dissemination. It is hoped that this will facilitate the development of evidence based guidelines for the management of major trauma. On the basis of the most recent data, MTOS participating hospitals have some cause for optimism. Between 1988 and 1996 the overall mortality ratio (the observed number of deaths divided by the expected number of deaths times · 100) has improved from 124 to 97. Over the 7-year period 1989-1995, after severity of injury is controlled for, the odds of death in children and young adults (<24 years) after severe injury declined by 16% a year [30]. It is not possible to identify, with certainty, which of the many facets of trauma patient management have contributed to this apparent improvement in outcome. However, it is very likely that developments in improved education, assessment and resuscitation techniques are major factors. One certain fact is that the proportion of seriously injured patients seen first by consultants or senior registrars has increased from 17% in 1988 to 30% in 1995 [29].

Quality assurance

Quality assurance is the process of assessment of performance of the delivery of care. The Trauma Anaesthesia Service should aim to ensure that high standards of clinical practice are maintained, both by individuals and the service as a whole. This will require assessment of the quality and appropriateness of patient care and identification, introduction and monitoring of essential developments. A specialist should be identified to oversee the quality assurance process.

Financial implications

By centralising skills, equipment and facility, trauma centres evolved as a cost limiting exercise. However a large proportion of trauma victims, particularly those with penetrating trauma, do not carry health insurance and government reimbursement for insured trauma patients often underestimates the actual costs incurred. The initial over expansion of trauma facilities in the USA led to a surplus and the recent closure of several centres.

Many factors must be taken into consideration when estimating the financial implications of trauma. These include medical expenses such as EMS costs, wage and productivity losses, administrative expenses (which include the administrative costs of private and public insurance plus police and legal costs), damage to property and goods, employer costs (representing the financial value incurred by remaining or newly trained workers), and the costs arising from both fatal and non-fatal injuries. Estimated in this way, the financial impact of trauma is immense. In the US in 1995, the costs arising from unintentional injuries alone were estimated to be $434.8 billion [31]. Such economic costs provide a measure of productivity lost and expenses incurred because of unintentional injuries. Economic costs, however, should not be used for cost benefit analysis because they do not reflect what society is willing to pay to prevent a fatality or injury. Comprehensive costs include not only the economic cost components, but also a measure of the value of lost quality of life associated with the deaths and injuries, that is, what society is willing to pay to prevent them. The values of lost quality of life can be estimated through empirical studies of what people actually pay to reduce their health and safety risks, such as through the purchase of air-bags or smoke detectors. In 1995 in the US, such lost quality of life was estimated to have a value of $775.8 billion, making the comprehensive cost of unintentional injury in the US $1,210.6 billion.

A comprehensive Trauma System is expensive, as is the provision of an appropriately staffed Trauma Anaesthesia Service. For example, the Trauma Anaesthesia Service of the Ryder Trauma Center provides a 24 h service to a specialist facility offering state of the art trauma care (Table 11). The Ryder Trauma Center admits 3 500-4 000 patients a year with 55% the result of blunt trauma and 45% the result of penetrating trauma. The operating rooms at the Ryder Center deal with 5 400 patients per year of which 2 500 are primary trauma patients. The estimated physician costs of running this anaesthesia service, which is provided by seven full time specialists and 13 trainees, is around $2,000,000.

Ensuring that adequate funding is available to provide this level of service has proved a major challenge. Suggested methods of increasing funding include the liquidation of illicit drug traffic assets for those suffering drug related trauma, and compensation schemes largely funded by employers. In Austria, the whole trauma system survives because employers pay 1.4% of total employee wages into the trauma system. Elsewhere in the world, it is usual for inadequate government funding to be supplemented by charitable contributions or reliance on funding from other services.

Table 11. The Ryder Trauma Center facility

Rooms/Beds	N
Trauma resuscitation rooms	5
Trauma resuscitation observation beds	6
Trauma operating rooms	6
Post-anaesthesia care unit beds	15
Trauma intensive care unit beds	20
Burn intensive care unit beds	5
Intermediate care unit beds	10
Regular ward beds	120

As dramatic as the financial costs may seem, the ultimate tragedy is not financial but personal. The loss experienced by victims and their families is incalculable. The primary solution to reducing the costs of trauma lies not in improved diagnostic and therapeutic efficiency, nor in financial wizardry or major overhauls in the organisation of trauma care systems, but in the prevention of trauma.

Prevention of trauma

Trauma is a major cause of death, disability and injury across the world. It's impact on society is enormous. Trauma eliminates a population of it's young men and women and accounts for many years of potential life lost. There are huge financial implications for countries with respect to both the acute medical costs, and to the loss of life of young people who would otherwise have been productive members of society.

While attention in recent years has been focused on establishing systems of management that allow faster, more efficient and higher quality care for the trauma victim to reduce deaths from trauma, it is clear that the most effective means of reducing trauma morbidity and mortality lies in prevention. Thirty years ago injuries were virtually ignored by the public health community. Their epidemiology was a mystery and few were advocating their prevention through research. Today the word "unintentional" is preferred to "accidental" because it is now recognised that many types of trauma are not just chance occurrences but are in fact quite predictable and therefore preventable. This has resulted in several laws that have led to a reduction in injuries from certain types of trauma. Motor vehicle related trauma has come under intense scrutiny. Laws concerning alcohol consumption, laminated windshields, energy absorbing steering wheels, crash resistant fuel systems, seat belts and most recently air-bags have all had a major impact on deaths and injury in motor vehicles. However, some of these advances have created their own problems; for example, the series of case reports of children being killed during airbag deployment [32].

The scope for trauma prevention is enormous. In the US, three particular areas have been highlighted that demand urgent changes in order to further reduce injury [33]. These are firearm legislation, speed limit controls and correct child occupant restraint in cars. To this should also be added the problem of illicit drug use that is particularly associated with penetrating trauma. It is clear that these are just a few of many strategies that could prevent injuries and deaths from trauma. As a prominent trauma clinician, the trauma anaesthetist has a major role to play in planning preventative strategies.

Conclusions

Trauma continues to be the most common cause of death in the first four decades of life and is a major cause of morbidity world-wide. It is clear that maximising survival in trauma victims requires definitive care as soon as possible and high quali-

Table 12. The ideal Trauma Anaesthesia Service

- Supported by a high quality facility and system
- Staffed by enthusiasts with adequate training
- Follow protocols but not restricted by them
- See enough patients to maintain skills but not burn out
- Adequate rest and reimbursement
- At the forefront of education and research
- Producing excellent results

ty care for all links in the trauma chain. The trauma anaesthetist has many skills essential to this process and has an important role to play in all phases of trauma care. As part of a multidisciplinary team, the trauma anaesthetist must strive to reduce this mortality. The provision of appropriate facilities and resources will lead to the development of high quality Trauma Anaesthesia Services (Table 12).

References

1. Royal College of Surgeons of England (1988) Report of the working party on the management of patients with major injuries. RCSE, London
2. Anderson ID, Woodford M, de Dombal T, Irving M (1988) A retrospective study of 1000 deaths from injury in England and Wales. Br Med J 296:1305-1308
3. Hussain LM, Redmond AD (1994) Are pre-hospital deaths from accidental injury preventable? Br Med J 308:1077-80
4. American College of Surgeons Committee on Trauma (1990) Hospital and pre-hospital resources for optimal care of the injured patient. Bull Am Coll Surg 77:20-29
5. Simpson HK, Smith GB (1996) Survey of paramedic skills in the United Kingdom and Channel Islands. Br Med J 313:1052-1053
6. Carli PA, Riou B, Barriot P (1993) France. In: Grande C (ed) Textbook of trauma anesthesia and critical care. Mosby-Year Book, St Louis, pp 199-204
7. Kaweski SM, Sise MJ, Virgilio RW (1990) The effect of pre-hospital fluids on survival in trauma patients. J Trauma 30:1215-1219
8. Potter D, Goldstein G, Fung SC, Selig M (1988) A controlled trial of pre-hospital advanced life support in trauma. Ann Emerg Med 17:582-588
9. Sampalis JS, Boukas S, Lavoie A, Nikolis A, Frechette P, Brown R, Fleiszer D, Mulder D (1995) Preventable death evaluation of the appropriateness of the on-site trauma care provided by Urgences-Sante physicians. J Trauma 39:1029-1035
10. Sampalis JS, Lavoie A, Williams JI, Mulder DS, Kalina M (1993) Impact of on-site care, pre-hospital time, and level of in-hospital care on survival in severely injured patients. J Trauma 34:252-261
11. Schmidt U, Frame SB, Nerlich ML, Rowe DW, Enderson BL, Maull KI, Tscherne H (1992) On-scene helicopter transport of patients with multiple injuries: comparison of a German and an American system. J Trauma 33:548-555
12. Smith JP, Bodai BL, Hill AS, Frey CF (1985) Pre-hospital stabilisation of critically injured patients: a failed concept. J Trauma 25:65-70
13. Cayten CG, Murphy JG, Stahl WM (1993) Basic life support versus advanced life support for injured patients with an injury severity score of 10 or more. J Trauma 35:460-467

14. Task Force of the American Heart Association, the European Resuscitation Council, the Heart and Stroke Foundation of Canada, and the Australian Resuscitation Council (1991) Recommended guidelines for uniform reporting of data from out of hospital cardiac arrest: the Utstein style. Circulation 84:960-975

15. Mackenzie CF, Nolan J, Kahn R, Delaney PA, Grande C (1996) Trauma anesthesia practices, training and facilities. Anesthesiology 85:A252

16. Cheng EY, Nimphius N, Kampine JP (1992) Anesthetic drugs and emergency departments. Anesth Analg 74:272-275

17. Oakley PA (1994) Setting and living up to national standards for the care of the injured. Injury 25:595-604

18. Rady MY (1994) Possible mechanisms for the interaction of peripheral somatic nerve stimulation, tissue injury, and hemorrhage in the pathophysiology of traumatic shock. Anesth Analg 78:761-765

19. Working Party of the Neuroanaesthesia Society of Great Britain and Ireland and the Association of Anaesthetists of Great Britain and Ireland (1996) Recommendations for the transfer of patients with acute head injuries to neurosurgical units. The Association of Anaesthetists of Great Britain and Ireland, London

20. Grande CM (ed) (1993) Textbook of trauma anesthesia and critical care. Mosby-Year Book, St Louis

21. Committee on Trauma of the American College of Surgeons (1989-1997) Advanced Trauma Life Support manual. American College of Surgeons, Chicago, IL

22. Ali J, Adam R, Butler AK et al (1993) Trauma outcome improves following the advanced trauma life support program in a developing country. J Trauma 34:890-898

23. Ali J, Adam R, Stedman M, Howard M, Williams JI (1994) Advanced trauma life support program increases emergency room application of trauma resuscitative procedures in a developing country. J Trauma 36:391-394

24. Bennett JR, Bodenham AR, Berridge JC (1992) Advanced trauma life support. A time for reappraisal. Anaesthesia 47:798-800

25. Mackenzie CF (1993) Simulation of trauma anaesthesia. In: Grande C (ed) Textbook of trauma anesthesia and critical care. Mosby-Year Book, St. Louis, pp 199-204

26. Wardrope J, Cross SF, Fothergill DJ (1990) One year's experience of major trauma outcome study methodology. Br Med J 301:156-159

27. Champion HR, Copes WS, Sacco WJ, Lawnick MM et al (1990) The major trauma outcome study: establishing national norms for trauma care. J Trauma 30:1356-1365

28. Yates DW, Woodford M, Hollis S (1992) Preliminary analysis of the care of injured patients in 33 British hospitals: first report of the United Kingdom major trauma outcome study. Br Med J 305:737-740

29. The UK Trauma Audit and Research Network (1996) A guide for clinicians. The University of Manchester, Manchester

30. Roberts I, Campbell F, Hollis S, Yates D (1996) On behalf of the Steering Committee of the Major Trauma Outcome Study Group. Reducing accident death rates in children and young adults: the contribution of hospital care. Br Med J 313:1239-1241

31. National Safety Council (1996) Accident Facts. National Safety Council, Itasca

32. Centers for Disease Control and Prevention (1997) Leads from the morbidity and mortality weekly report. Update: fatal air bag-related injuries children.JAMA 277(1):11-12

33. Baker SP (1997) Advances and adventures in trauma prevention. J Trauma 42:369-373

Chapter 15

Anaesthetic implications of drug abuse in trauma patients

M.J.A. Parr, R.J.H. Hadfield

It is increasingly recognised that drug abuse not only contributes to the trauma patient population but also that the effects of acute and chronic drug toxicity have major implications for patient management. The role of drug abuse as a factor associated with morbidity and mortality in the trauma setting has not been properly quantified. Physicians dealing with victims of acute trauma will however, inevitably have to deal with the associated problems of drug abuse. For optimal management of these patients a thorough working knowledge of commonly abused drugs is required.

United Nations estimates suggest that drug trafficking accounts for at least 10% of all international trade, with an annual net worth of more than $480 billion. Cannabis is the most common drug used throughout the world with more that 140 million habitual smokers (>2.5% of the world population). Synthetic drugs particularly amphetamines, amphetamine derivatives and LSD are the next most common group of drugs abused followed by cocaine, heroin and other opioids.

In the UK the number of drug addicts notified to the Home Office for the 6 months ending March 1996 increased by 2% to 23 313, a slightly smaller increase than in recent years [1]. These notification rates are generally accepted to represent only around 20% of actual addicts, and therefore represent only the crudest of estimates. The ratio of males to females remains 3:1. Over half the users presenting are in their twenties and more than 10% are between 15 and 19 years old. Some 54% of users reported heroin as their main drug, an increase from 52% in the previous period. Methadone and amphetamine continue to be the next most frequently reported main drugs abused, at 15% and 10% respectively. Cocaine was the main drug abused by only 4% which contrasts markedly with US experience . It is estimated that there are more than 50 million drug abusers world-wide. According to the United Nations Drug Control Programme, European seizures in 1992 included 18.2 tonnes of cocaine and 7.2 tonnes of heroin. It is clear therefore that the scale of the problem is enormous.

The United States has appreciated the extent of their drug problem for longer than many and consequently has better information than most other countries. While the US experience does not automatically translate to other countries there is a lot to be learnt from the information that is available. Alcohol has been implicated consistently in more than 50% of trauma deaths and the Insurance Institute for Highway Safety usually reports alcohol is detected in 70% of fatally injured drivers. Of more recent concern is the increasing evidence that illicit drug abuse is playing a major role in the production of trauma and crime. In a paper from

Knoxville looking at 201 injured drivers over a 5 month period admitted to a level 1 trauma centre, Kirby found 37% had positive blood alcohol concentrations (BAC), while 40% tested positive for other drugs. More than half of the drivers using alcohol also had other drugs detected [2]. Lindenbaum and colleagues looking at an urban trauma population, assessed 169 trauma cases over a 9 month period. They found 52% tested positive for cocaine, 37% were positive for cannabinoids, alcohol was present in 35% and that violent crime was associated with a positive drug screen in 80% of cases [3]. Unfortunately the finding of a negative drug screen on testing does not necessarily exclude drug dependence. Soderstrom found substance dependence in 69% of patients who were tested negative on admission to a Baltimore trauma centre [4].

While the problem in the UK and many other countries is not on the same scale as the USA we share a common need with our American colleagues. A recent news release from the Department of Transport states that preliminary evidence from the first 7 months of a 3-year survey suggest that illicit drug taking by road accident victims (drivers, passengers, riders and pedestrians) has increased fourfold, more than one drug is increasingly found and the presence of alcohol has fallen substantially [5].

This discussion will concentrate on the most common drugs encountered in the trauma setting; these are cocaine, narcotics, marijuana, amphetamine derivatives, benzodiazepines, LSD and phencyclidine.

Common principles

When dealing with the effects of drug abuse a number of common principles can be identified.
1. Drug histories are usually unavailable or unreliable, either because the patient is concerned about litigation or because they are unable to give a history.
2. For the major trauma patient with cardiovascular, respiratory and neurological depression differentiating the effects of intoxication from the effects of trauma can be extremely difficult.
3. The neurological sequelae of acute drug intoxication in particular can pose a major problem. The disorientated, agitated, aggressive, stuporous or comatose patient presents multiple difficulties in assessment and management. The differential diagnosis includes intracranial pathology (focal or diffuse, primary or secondary), metabolic causes and the direct effects of drugs. There may be problems starting lines, keeping an oxygen mask on, and performing X-rays.
4. An aggressive policy of rapid sequence induction, endotracheal intubation and the rapid exclusion of these causes in this group of patients may be the safest option. This avoids the patient injuring themselves or the trauma team, reduces the chance of secondary brain injury, and makes anaesthesia/surgical conditions optimal for any intervention that is needed.
5. Failure to identify correctable intracranial pathology can be devastating and it is unwise to assume a depressed level of consciousness is due to drug intoxication in trauma patients [6].

6. Multiple drug abuse is common with an increased potential for tolerance, interaction and delayed effects. Tolerance develops as a result of enzyme induction and/or receptor adaptation and cross tolerance may effect a number of other drugs. There is a high potential for drug interactions, and as well as the effects of the illicit drugs there is a need to remember the possibility of adulterants. To confuse the issue quinine, strychnine, local anaesthetics, and sugars are often used by the more knowledgeable dealers while baking soda and talc are used by the less discriminating. "Body packing", the art of drug smuggling in various body orifices, may result in contamination by enteric bacteria and subsequent sepsis in the user.
7. The high standards of monitoring common to the management of trauma patients should be maintained and admission to a high dependency/intensive care facility to achieve this is often appropriate.
8. Despite the huge numbers of different illicit drugs with a variety of actions it is fortunate that the common principles of general management remain the same: to secure the airway, maintain adequate ventilation and ensure effective oxygen delivery to the tissues. The use of specific antidotes in the trauma setting is limited.

Cocaine

By 1986 it was estimated that almost 15% of the US population had tried cocaine, with nearly 40% in the age range of 25-30 years [7]. In the United States it is now the number one cause for drug-related emergency department visits in urban settings. An estimated 25 million Americans have used it at least once, 5 million use it regularly, and >250 000 are addicted. Fatal injury associated with cocaine use is now recognised as the most common cause of death in young adult males in New York city, with 66% of deaths due to trauma and 33% due to toxicity. Cocaine metabolites are detectable in 26% of NYC residents suffering fatal injury [8]. Although the mechanisms of cocaine toxicity are not well understood, the drug can affect nearly every organ system.

Cocaine is an ester of benzoic acid and has a plasma half-life of 90 min but tachyphylaxis results in a euphoretic half-life of around 45 min. Psychiatric symptoms vary among stimulant abusers and within an abuser over time. Accidents, illegal acts and atypical sexual behaviour occur in more than 80% of regular cocaine users (Table 1).

Originally an expensive recreational drug of the rich, cocaine has now become cheap and readily available. Administration is by any route imaginable but it is most commonly snorted or smoked. Cocaine is available in two forms: cocaine hydrochloride, which is usually taken by snorting or injection, and "crack" cocaine, which is smoked. After snorting blood levels reach a peak at 1 h and most is metabolised within 2-3 h. Freebase or crack cocaine has been widely available since 1984. Crack cocaine can be vaporised (melting point 98°C) and inhaled as smoke. The name "crack" is derived from the noise the crystals make while being

Table 1. Neuropsychiatric effects of cocaine intoxication

• Disinihibition	• Psychosis
• Impaired judgement	• Delerium
• Grandiosity	• Convulsions
• Impulsiveness	• Vascular headache
• Hypersexuality	• Cerebral vasculitis
• Hypervigilance	• Cerebral ischaemia and infarction
• Compulsive actions	• Cerebral haemorrhage
• Extreme psychomotor activation	• Cerebral oedema
• Tremors	

heated. Cocaine which is smoked or injected intravenously produces peak serum concentrations in 5-15 min with a half-life of 30-45 min.

The active substance in cocaine is methylbenzoylecgonine which has a relatively large volume of distribution and is metabolised via hepatic and plasma esterases. Cocaine in small amounts is detectable in urine for 3-6 h post-administration, but metabolites (i.e., benzoylecgonine) can be detected for 14-60 h.

The action of cocaine on sodium channels results in the local anaesthetic action on peripheral nerves. The systemic effects of cocaine are due to inhibition of norepinephrine re-uptake at peripheral sympathetic nerve endings and the inhibition of norepinephrine and dopamine re-uptake at central presynaptic sites. The result is postsynaptic accumulation of catecholamines with increased sympathetic effects.

The medical complications associated with cocaine abuse range from single organ system involvement to death. Most cocaine fatalities are due to seizures, stroke, cardiac arrhythmia or myocardial infarction which may be seen in otherwise healthy normal individuals. Although many fatalities related to cocaine have a close temporal relationship to administration, up to a third will not occur until 6-24 h later.

The cardiovascular effects of cocaine are diverse (Table 2). The sclerosis of vessels follows repeated injection and is common to all injectable drugs. However as cocaine is a vasoconstrictor it is more likely to cause vascular problems. As the user runs out of peripheral veins they may use central access or opt for other routes, for example skin popping that produces characteristic scarring.

There are over 100 cases of acute myocardial infarction reported in the literature on cocaine. Some 70% of victims have no cardiac history and 90% are young

Table 2. Cardiovascular complications of cocaine abuse

• Vessel sclerosis	• Cardiomyopathy
• Hypertension	• Cerebral infarction and haemorrhage
• Tachyarrhythmias	• Aortic rupture
• Myocardial ischaemia and infarction	• Bowel ischaemia and infarction
• Myocarditis	

males who are regular cocaine snorters. However it may occur on the first exposure to the drug within minutes or up to 15 h after cocaine use and is not frequency, dose or route related. Coronary thrombosis is seen in association with coronary vasoconstriction at a time when myocardial oxygen demand is increased by the sympathetic effects of cocaine. Accelerated atherosclerosis (which is reproducible in rabbits) is recognised in some cases while others show complete thrombotic occlusion of normal vessels [9]. Cocaine increases platelet aggregation by α-granule release and fibrinogen binding and may also induce an endovascular injury and procoagulatory state.

Other cardiovascular effects of cocaine toxicity include myocarditis [10], aortic rupture [11]; chronic ST-T elevation has been noted in long-term cocaine users. A dilated cardiomyopathy, which appears to resemble the myocardial dysfunction of phaeochromocytoma or chronic amphetamine abuse and improves with avoidance of further cocaine use, has recently been described [12].

Asymptomatic coronary vasoconstriction with a 33% increase in coronary artery resistance has been demonstrated in response to 2 mg/kg intranasal cocaine in patients having coronary angiography. The coronary vasospasm was reversed by intracoronary phentolamine (total dose of 2 mg), demonstrating it is an α-sympathomimetic effect [13]. Cardiac arrhythmias that are blamed for many out of hospital cocaine deaths include supraventricular tachycardia, ventricular tachycardia and ventricular fibrillation [14]. The treatment of these arrhythmias with β-blockers has brought to light an important effect in that β-blockade alone may result in unopposed α-activity and increased coronary vasoconstriction and hypertension [15, 16]. Therefore the current recommendation for blocking the sympathomimetic effects of cocaine is to use an agent with some α-blockade (i.e., labetolol), or a selective β-1 agent (i.e., esmolol) [17-19]. When significant ventricular arrhythmias occur, lignocaine has been used with some success. However, lignocaine exerts its antiarrhythmic properties by inhibiting fast sodium channels similar to the effect of cocaine. Therefore, it is possible that lignocaine could aggravate the toxicity of cocaine [20]. The use of lignocaine to control ventricular arrhythmias may also potentiate cocaine induced seizures and lower the seizure threshold.

There are numerous respiratory complications that are associated with cocaine abuse (Table 3). The toxic effects on the lungs depend upon the route of administration [21]. Barotrauma arises from the forceful Valsalva manoeuvres that are done during smoking and may easily be confused with barotrauma resulting from the effects of trauma [22]. Pulmonary haemorrhage has been found in cocaine smokers which may also be confused with thoracic trauma. Usually this is an occult finding on biopsy or autopsy but massive haemoptysis may be seen occasionally. Bronchiolitis obliterans organising pneumonia [23] and "crack lung", characterised by bronchospasm, fever, and transient pulmonary infiltrates, have also been described. Eosinophilia and elevated serum IgE levels lend support to the belief that this is a hypersensitivity reaction. Pulmonary oedema may have a multifactorial aetiology. A hydrostatic leak may result from cardiogenic failure or large negative intrathoracic pressures during inhalation. A capillary leak may result from a cocaine induced microangiopathy or immunogenic causes with resultant pulmonary oedema in the presence of normal myocardial function [24].

Table 3. Pulmonary effects of cocaine abuse

- Nasal perforation
- Barotrauma
- Black sputum bronchitis
- Pulmonary haemorrhage
- Pulmonary oedema
- Pulmonary hypertension
- Granulomatous pneumonitis
- Bronchiolitis obliterating organising pneumonia (BOOP)

Altered mental states at the time of Emergency Department presentation may be seen in up to 37% of cocaine abusers [25]. Cocaine causes both ischaemic and haemorrhage strokes [26] and subarachnoid haemorrhage [27]. Neurological episodes are ischaemic in 54% of cases and haemorrhage in 46%, the overall mortality is 6% if patients exhibit focal neurological signs [28]. When this was first recognised, it was usually associated with an underlying berry aneurysm or arteriovenous malformation and it was suggested that cocaine caused severe hypertension, leading to rupture at a site of underlying vascular weakness. More recently, subarachnoid haemorrhage has been recognised in the absence of vascular malformations prompting speculation that cocaine causes a form of vasculitis [29].

The most common major CNS toxicity associated with cocaine use is generalised seizures [30]. Seizures may result from focal bleeds or ischaemic or direct toxicity as cocaine like the other local anaesthetics reduces the seizure threshold. In some animal models the long-term repeated administration of cocaine results in a progressive lowering of the seizure threshold. Seizures may eventually occur spontaneously, in the absence of further cocaine administration.

Miscellaneous effects of cocaine abuse include nausea, vomiting, hyperpyrexia, rhabdomyolysis, disseminated intravascular coagulation, acute renal failure, hepatitis and increased anaesthetic requirements. Cocaine induced rhabdomyolysis has been seen in association with hyperpyrexia [31]. The high serum creatine phosphokinase (CPK) level may be difficult to interpret in the presence of multiple trauma. The mechanism of cocaine-induced rhabdomyolysis is unclear but may be due to muscular overexertion, ischaemia of skeletal muscles or a direct toxic injury to the myocyte. Cocaine associated hepatitis has been described [32]. Increased anaesthetic requirements may be expected because of the arousal effects of cocaine. A dose dependent increase in minimum anaesthetic concentration (MAC) with increasing cocaine administration has been demonstrated in animal models [33]. The effect peaked 3 h after IV infusion and had returned to normal by 24 h.

The pregnant intoxicated traumatised patient is a well recognised problem in urban America. There are now two patients to consider, as the issue is made increasingly difficult because cocaine intoxication can produce signs and symptoms that are impossible to differentiate from the effects of pre-eclampsia [24]. In one study from the US, 14% of delivery patients tested positive for cocaine [34]. In addition, cocaine use is associated with abruptio placentae, spontaneous abortion, pre-term labour, foetal abnormalities and "crack babies". Cocaine causes constriction of uterine vascular beds with resultant placental ischaemia and has been implicated in myocardial and cerebral infarction in the foetus [35].

There is no specific antidote to counteract the general toxicity or the multisystem complications of cocaine abuse. Supportive measures are the mainstay of treatment. The one pharmacologic agent which has most consistently shown protective and therapeutic benefits in the general management of these patients is diazepam [36]. It helps prevent hyperthermia, acidaemia, agitation and seizures and moderates the cardiovascular responses to cocaine.

Narcotics

The acute neurological effects of narcotics are familiar to all anaesthetists and emergency physicians (Table 4). The acute use of narcotics reduces the requirement for anaesthesia however, the chronic use results in tolerance and in an increase in anaesthetic/analgesic requirement. The triad of coma, respiratory depression and miotic pupils suggests opioid intoxication. Respiratory depression causing hypoxia is the major threat to life. Mydriasis and convulsions, if they occur, are most commonly due to hypoxia. Convulsions may rarely occur with the accumulation of normeperidine, the neurotoxic metabolite of meperidine [37, 38].

The cardiovascular effects of narcotic abuse include sclerosis of peripheral and central vessels following injection, orthostatic hypotension, syncope, myocardial depression, valve lesions, endocarditis and the transmission of blood borne infection.

The pulmonary complications arise due to respiratory depression and sepsis and again barotrauma is seen in smokers. Recognised complications include recurrent pneumonias, septic emboli, aspiration pneumonitis, atelectasis, pulmonary oedema and pulmonary hypertension. Opioid induced noncardiogenic pulmonary oedema is most commonly seen following heroin overdose but has been reported after overdoses with most opioids [39]. The pulmonary oedema is thought to be

Table 4. Effects of narcotic

- Analgesia
- Mood change
- Drowsiness
- Euphoria
- Nausea
- Vomiting
- Respiratory depression
- Miosis

produced by altered permeability of the pulmonary capillaries that is mediated by the opioid. Rhabdomyolysis may occur secondary to immobility following overdose or possibly through a direct effect of the opioid, again in the trauma setting this will be difficult to interpret.

Septic complications can be local or generalised and are usually the cause of death in the chronic abusers that manage to avoid trauma. Infective complications include superficial infections at the site of injection, septicaemia, bacterial endocarditis, hepatitis B, hepatitis C and HIV. Infective complications are common to all intravenous abusers but not confined to this route of exposure; chronic abuse of a variety of drugs by a variety of routes is associated with immune deficiency and behaviour that is likely to put the abuser at risk of hepatitis and HIV. From a study of 2523 patients attending an Emergency Department in Baltimore in 1992, 5% were hepatitis B positive, 18% hepatitis C positive and 6% HIV positive. In many US trauma centres the majority of penetrating trauma victims are HIV positive and HIV is now the leading cause of death in American males between the ages of 25 and 44 years [40].

Heroin is currently the street favourite in the UK and many other countries because of the "rush" it generates. Heroin is rapidly metabolised to 6-monoacetylmorphine and then metabolised to morphine by the liver. Toxicity is therefore primarily related to morphine and various adulterants. Street heroin in the UK ranges in purity from 10% to 80% and accounts for 200 deaths per annum, from aspiration, respiratory depression and pulmonary oedema. The impact of heroin in the trauma population is unknown at present.

Methadone is a synthetic opioid widely used for opioid detoxification and maintenance therapy and consequently is widely available for abuse. Methadone is used for detoxification primarily because of the absence of significant euphoria and its long half-life of 15-25 h.

Naloxone is the specific antidote of choice. It has pure antagonist properties at all clinically important opioid receptors [41] and a half-life of approximately 60 min, whereas the half-lives of most opioid agonists are longer. Routes of administration include intravenous, intramuscular, subcutaneous, and tracheal [42]. The role of naloxone in the trauma setting is limited. It should not be administered if significant head injury is suspected. The adverse effects of naloxone on haemodynamics and ICP (intra-cranial pressure) and the risk of producing an agitated uncontrollable patient means that it has little role to play in the acute trauma resuscitation setting. Equally the risks of producing a narcotic withdrawal syndrome and depriving an injured patient of analgesia should be borne in mind.

Narcotic withdrawal results in a characteristic withdrawal syndrome ("cold turkey") (Table 5). Opioid withdrawal is not usually life-threatening to the adult patient and although extremely unpleasant can often be tolerated without pharmacologic intervention [43]. Clonidine, an α-2 agonist, has been used to modulate the symptoms of opioid withdrawal [44]. Clonidine however, is also available for illicit use as it is said to boost the effect of methadone. Abrupt clonidine withdrawal is also associated with a withdrawal syndrome and if being abused should be withdrawn slowly. Unlike the adult, narcotic withdrawal in newborn infants is potentially life-threatening [45]. Irritability, tremors, high-pitched cry, and incon-

Table 5. Narcotic withdrawal syndrome "cold turkey"

• Agitation	• Dilated pupils
• Craving	• Hypertension
• Anorexia	• Tachycardia
• Anxiety	• Piloerection
• Nausea	• Lacrimation
• Vomiting	• Rhinorrhea
• Muscle and bone aches	• Fever
• Diarrhoea	• Sweating

solablity are signs of an opioid dependent infant. Symptoms usually start within 48 h of birth and seizures represent the largest threat to life. Narcotic withdrawal has also been reported to cause tachycardia and hypotension, with failure to respond to vasoactive agents; this is however, rarely seen in the trauma anaesthesia setting as they are corrected by opioid administration. Higher than usual narcotic doses are to be expected in these patients. Regional blocks and epidurals are an excellent alternative to the often large doses of narcotics that make pharmacy and nursing staff very nervous. Manipulative drug seeking behaviour is to be expected.

Marijuana

The Indian hemp plant (*Cannabis sativa*) contain numerous compounds collectively referred to as cannabinoids. The major psychotropic compound is Δ^9-tetrahydrocannabinol (THC) which is rapidly absorbed from the respiratory and gastrointestinal mucosa. Peak plasma levels of THC are reached within 10 min of smoking and 45 min of oral ingestion. THC is metabolised by the liver with predominant excretion in the urine. Marijuana produces mild alterations in mood, sensory perception, and co-ordination.

The effects of marijuana can be very variable. In general marijuana stimulates the sympathetic nervous system and inhibits the parasympathetic system with a duration of effect lasting 2-3 h after smoking and 3-5 h after ingestion. Mild elevations in vital signs may be seen with increases in heart rate and cardiac output. Trauma related to perceptual alterations are the most serious risks to life. Congestion of conjunctival blood vessels leading to reddened conjunctiva is a highly sensitive but not specific indicator of recent marijuana use. In volunteers, THC enhanced the respiratory depressant effects of oxymorphone and pentobarbital and also potentiated the neurological and cardiovascular effects of alcohol [46]. Marijuana reduces anaesthetic requirements in dogs, with the effect not persisting beyond 3 h post-administration [47].

Amphetamines

The phenylethylamine structure provides the basis for the synthesis of a wide range of neurotransmitters. Substitution of methoxyl groups leads to several synthetic hallucinogenic amphetamines. Because these drugs are not naturally occurring they have been labelled as "designer drugs". Amphetamines increase the release and reduce re-uptake of catecholamines at nerve endings producing alertness that increases anaesthetic requirement. Dextroamphetamine administered to animals increases MAC in a dose dependent manner. Their effect is therefore similar to that of cocaine with features of intoxication including anxiety, psychosis, convulsions, mydriasis and hypertensive encephalopathy. Myocardial ischaemia and infarction, serious arrhythmias, hyperthermia, acidosis and necrotizing angiitis are also recognised. Prolonged use however, leads to catecholamine depletion more commonly than cocaine and their duration of effect is four to eight times that of cocaine. This may result in hypotension and bradycardia which is refractory to the use of indirect pressors such as ephedrine. Small titrated amounts of direct-acting catecholamines such as epinephrine or norepinephrine may be required to maintain cardiovascular stability.

Amphetamine use is on the decrease, largely because of the unpleasant side effects and the ready availability and cheapness of alternatives. In the UK use of amphetamine derivatives, in particular "ecstasy" (3.4 methylenedioxymethamphetamine, MDMA) has reached epidemic proportions with estimates that more than a million tablets are ingested every week. Ecstasy intoxication and the results of its use lead to diverse clinical presentations of life threatening complications (Table 6). In a recent study of teenagers in the northwest of England, half had tried drugs by the age of 16 years [48]. It is now estimated that 7.3% of girls and 9.2% of boys in the 15-16 year old age group have experimented with MDMA [49]. This represents a large increase on estimates from 1989 when the level of experimentation in the 16 year old age group was 2% [50].

The pharmacological basis for the actions of MDMA appears to be centred around serotonin transport [51]. Amphetamine derivatives have been shown to cause an initial release of serotonin both in vitro [52, 53] and in vivo [54-56] followed by a more long term depletion of serotonin which may last for several

Table 6. Life threatening complications associated with MDMA ingestion

• Hyperthermia	• Arrhythmias
• Coagulopathy (DIC)	• Hypertension
• Rhabdomyolysis	• Hypotension
• Renal failure	• Seizures
• Acidosis	• Coma
• Hyperkalaemia	• Intracranial infarction and thrombosis
• Hepatic failure	• Intracranial haemorrhage
• Hypoglycaemia	• Trauma
• Hyponatraemia	• Neuropsychiatric disorders

months [57, 58]. Acute stimulation of serotonin and dopaminergic systems results in an increased release of neurotransmitters with a predominant sympathomimetic effect demonstrated by hypertension, tachycardia, arrhythmias, sweating and pupillary dilatation [59].

MDMA intoxication has been recognised in association with major trauma [60-62]. However it is likely that many individuals with traumatic injuries have been treated and anaesthetised without knowledge of their MDMA intoxicated state. As with cocaine intoxication differentiating the sympathomimetic effects of intoxication from the sympathetic response to trauma and pain is not possible on clinical grounds. Hyperthermia is recognised as a complication of ecstasy abuse and may be confused with malignant hyperpyrexia (MH) if it occurs after the administration of MH trigger agents. Should a hyperpyrexic reaction occur during anaesthesia, confusion over the diagnosis is not a practical problem since in both cases the mainstay of treatment is control of body temperature with dantrolene, cooling and general supportive care [63]. Dantrolene may be of use in cases of drug induced hyperthermia, which include malignant hyperthermia, the malignant neuroleptic syndrome and intoxication with MDMA [64-67]. There have been no reported survivors with a temperature greater than 42°C and the degree of neurological deficit in survivors may be related to the peak temperature. In the absence of hyperpyrexia there would appear to be no role for dantrolene in the management of complications.

Benzodiazepines

The benzodiazepines are among the world's most widely prescribed drugs and consequently are freely available for abuse. They are often taken with other drugs and quite commonly in surprising mixtures with various stimulants. The actions of benzodiazepines are familiar to all anaesthetists and emergency physicians. Sedation ranging from drowsiness to coma with respiratory depression, cardiovascular depression with vasodilatation and hypothermia are the prominent features. Elimination half-life varies considerably for example, the ultra-short acting midazolam has a half-life of 2-5 h while diazepam is usually 20-50 h but in high dose abusers may be increased up to 94 h [68]. These drugs are highly protein bound, highly lipid soluble and most are eliminated by metabolism in the liver. Flumazenil, the specific benzodiazepine antagonist, is widely distributed in the tissues and has a high hepatic clearance. The plasma half-life of 0.7-1.3 h for flumazenil is clearly shorter than the half-life of most benzodiazepines. In the context of trauma flumazenil should be used with caution because of associated adverse effects which include: the unmasking effect of proconvulsant drug, the production of a withdrawal state in a dependent patient (with emergence delirium and induction of convulsions), incomplete reversal of respiratory depression, resedation because of the short half-life and increased sympathetic effects in a mixed overdose by removing the protective effect of benzodiazepines [69].

Lysergic acid diethylamide

Lysergic acid diethylamide (LSD) is a substituted indole alkylamine with a main effect of producing visual and auditory hallucinations through central serotonin modulation [70]. LSD has some analgesic action and may prolong the analgesic effects of narcotics. Its physical effects last 6-8 h and the psychic effects 12-18 h. Medical complications usually result from trauma related to the hallucinations. Flashbacks (repetition of previous hallucination even after prolonged drug free periods) have been precipitated by anaesthesia and traumatic events and are usually easily managed with benzodiazepines. Agitation, seizures and respiratory arrest have been known to occur in acute intoxication.

Phencyclidine

Phencyclidine (PCP) and ketamine represent a unique class of anaesthetic agents that result in dissociative anaesthesia and profound analgesia [71]. PCP has a terminal half-life of approximately 18-24 h and was removed from the pharmaceutical market in 1963 due to hallucinations, agitation, and muscle rigidity on emergence. Early oral abuse of PCP has been replace by smoking (often with marijuana) as this allows better titration of the effect and less severe side effects.

In low doses, mild stimulant effects may be seen, larger doses produce muscle rigidity, hallucinations and psychosis and high doses result in coma and seizures [72]. Violent behaviour and insensitivity to pain can be seen at any time and is not dose related. Horizontal nystagnus which may progress to vertical or rotary can be seen even in low doses and may be helpful in making a diagnosis [73]. PCPs behavioural effects leading to violence and trauma represent the largest threat to life. Less commonly dopaminergic storm, with hypertension, intracerebral bleeding and seizures, has also been seen.

General management

A number of general management principles apply when dealing with trauma patients who are drug abusers:
1. protect yourself from physical injury and infection. There is a high risk of blood borne infection and appropriate precautions include wearing eye protection, masks, fluid impermeable gowns and gloves;
2. carefully follow the ABC format for resuscitation;
3. keep an open mind and exclude physical or metabolic correctable causes for abnormalities before putting the blame on drug intoxication;
4. anticipate and protect the patient from the effects of acute drug intoxication, which requires monitoring the patient during the perioperative period, with psychological and physical assessment, Further monitoring is likely to include temperature, ECG, BP, pulse oximetry, serum biochemistry and blood gases;
5. perform appropriate drug screening tests;

6. anticipate the complications of chronic drug usage and take appropriate action;
7. anticipate withdrawal syndromes and start appropriate prophylactic treatment, avoid the use of antagonist drugs;
8. titrate anaesthetic, sedative and analgesic drugs;
9. use direct vasopressors as prolonged drug abuse may result in catecholamine depletion;
10. use drugs with short half lives, the instability of trauma patients leaves little role for long acting vasodepressors;
11. anticipate abnormal postoperative drug requirements;
12. arrange for access to detoxification and support services.

Conclusions

Illicit drug use is becoming an increasing problem in the trauma setting where failure to appreciate drug intoxication may well lead to adverse events and poor outcomes. A comprehensive working knowledge of the commonly abused drugs is therefore required for optimal management of these patients. There is also now an increasing recognition that death and injury as a result of alcohol and drug abuse are preventable, in that they are treatable conditions. Drug screening of individuals involved in accidents or causing injury is necessary to identify these individuals and will allow assessment of the true impact of illicit drug abuse on trauma morbidity and mortality. Preventative strategies through education are required and should receive a high priority.

References

1. Government Statistical Service (1997) Statistical bulletin. Department of Health, p 1
2. Kirby JM, Maull KI, Fain W (1992) Comparability of alcohol and drug use in injured drivers. Southern Med Journal 85:800-801
3. Lindenbaum GA, Carrol SF, Daskal I et al (1989) Patterns of alcohol and drug abuse in an urban trauma center: the increasing role of cocaine abuse. J Trauma 29:1654-1658
4. Soderstrom CA, Dischinger PC, Smith GS et al (1992) Psychoactive substance dependence among trauma center patients. JAMA 267:2756-2759
5. Department of Transport (1997) News release, press notice 149/Transport
6. Galbraith S (1976) Misdiagnosis and delayed diagnosis of traumatic intracranial haematoma. British Medical Journal 1:1438
7. Abelson HI, Miller JD (1985) A decade in trends in cocaine use in the household population. Nat Inst Drug Abuse Res Monogr Ser 61:35-49
8. Marzuk PM, Tardiff K, Leon AC et al (1995) Fatal injuries after cocaine use as a leading cause of death among young adults in New York City. N Eng J Med 26:1753
9. Pasternack PF, Colvin SE, Baumann FG (1985) Cocaine induced angina pectoris and myocardial infarction in patients younger than 40 years. Am J Cardiol 55:847
10. Isner JM, Estes M, Thompson PD et al (1986) Acute cardiac events temporarily related to cocaine abuse. N Engl J Med 315:1438
11. Barth CW, Bray M, Roberts WC (1986) Rupture of the ascending aorta during cocaine intoxication. Am J Cardiol 57:496

12. Chokshi SK, Moore R, Pondion NG et al (1989) Reversible cardiomyopathy associated with cocaine intoxication. Ann Intern Med 111:1039
13. Lange RA, Cigarroa RG, Yancy CW Jr et al (1989) Cocaine induced coronary artery vasoconstriction. N Eng J Med 321:1557-1562
14. Cregler LL, Mark H (1986) Cardiovascular dangers of cocaine abuse. Am J Cardiol 57:1185
15. Lange RA, Cigarroa RG, Flores ED et al (1990) Potentiation of cocaine-induced coronary vasoconstriction by beta-adrenergic blockade. Ann Intern Med 112:897-903
16. Ramoska E, Sacchetti AD (1985) Propranolol-induced hypertension in treatment of cocaine intoxication. Ann Emerg Med 14:1112
17. Gay GR, Loper KA (1988) The use of labetolol in the management of cocaine crisis. Ann Emerg Med 17:282-283
18. Dusenberry SJ, Hicks MJ, Mariani PJ (1987) Labetalol treatment of cocaine toxicity. Ann Emerg Med 16:235
19. Pollan S, Tadjziechy M (1989) Esmolol in the management of epinephrine and cocaine induced cardiovascular toxicity. Anesth Analg 69:663-664
20. Derlet RW, Albertson TE (1990) Potentiation of cocaine toxicity with lidocaine. Ann Emerg Med 19:464
21. Itkonen J, Schnoll S, Glassroth J (1984) Pulmonary dysfunction in "freebase" cocaine users. Arch Int Med 144:2195
22. Shesser R, Davis C, Edelsten S (1981) Pneumomediastinum and pneumothorax after inhaling alkaloidal cocaine. Ann Emerg Med 10:213
23. Patal RC, Dutta D, Schonfeld SA (1987) Free-base cocaine use associated with bronchiolitis obliterans organizing pneumonia. Ann Intern Med 107:186
24. Campbell D, Parr MJA, Shutt LE (1996) Unrecognised crack cocaine abuse in pregnancy. Br J Anaesthesia 77:553-555
25. Derlet RW, Albertson TE (1986) Emergency department presentation of cocaine intoxication. Ann Emerg Med 18:182
26. Seaman ME (1990) Acute cocaine abuse associated with cerebral infarction. Ann Emerg Med 19:34
27. Lichtenfeld PJ, Rubin DB, Feldman RS (1984) Subarachnoid hemorrhage precipitated by cocaine snorting. Arch Neurol 411:223
28. Peterson PL, Roszler M, Jacobs I et al (1991) Neurovascular complications of cocaine abuse. J Neuropsychiat Clin Neurosci 3:143
29. Kay BR, Fainstate M (1987) Cerebral vasculitis associated with cocaine abuse. JAMA 258:2104
30. Myers JA, Barnett MF (1984) Generalized seizures and cocaine abuse. Neurology 344:1675
31. Merigian KS, Roberts JR (1987) Cocaine intoxication: hyperyrexia, rhabdomyolysis, and acute renal failure. Clin Toxicol 25:135
32. Perinol LE, Warren GE, Levine JS (1987) Cocaine induced hepatoxicity in humans. Gastroenterology 93:176
33. Stoelting RK, Creassor CW, Martz RC (1975) Effects of cocaine on halothane MAC in dogs. Anesth Analg 54:422
34. Matera C, Warren WB, Moomjy M et al (1990) Prevalence of the use of cocaine and other substances in an obstetric population. Am J Obstet Gynecol 163:797
35. Woods JR, Plessinger MA, Clark KE (1987) Effect of cocaine on uterine blood flow and fetal oxygenation. JAMA 257:957
36. Derlet RW, Albertson TE (1989) Agents that protect against cocaine induced death and seizures. Ann Emerg Med 18:446

37. Goetting MG (1985) Neurotoxicity of meperidine. Ann Emerg Med 14:1007
38. Stone PA, MacIntyre PE, Jarvis DA (1993) Norpethidine toxicity and patient controlled analgesia. BJA 71:738-740
39. Duberstein JL, Kaufman DM (1971) A clinical study of an epidemic of heroin intoxication and heroin induced pulmonary oedema. Am J Med 51:704
40. National Safety Council (1996) Accident facts. National Safety Council, Itasca
41. Goldfrank LR (1984) The several uses of naloxone. Emerg Med 16:105
42. Tandberg D, Abercrombie D (1982) Treatment of heroin overdosage with endotracheal naloxone. Ann Emerg Med 11:443
43. George CF, Robertson D (1987) Clinical consequences of abrupt drug withdrawal. Med Toxicol 2:367
44. Gossop M (1988) Clonidine and the treatment of the opioid withdrawal syndrome. Drug Alcohol Depend 21:253
45. Sweet AY (1982) Narcotic withdrawal syndrome in the newborn. Pediatr Rev 3:285
46. Johnstone RE, Lief PL, Kulp RA et al (1975) Combination of delta-9-tetrahydrocannabinol with oxymorphone and pentobarbital. Anesthesiology 42:674
47. Stoelting RK, Martz RC, Gartner J et al (1973) Effects of delta-9-tetrahydrocannabinol on halothane MAC in dogs. Anesthesiology 38:521
48. Parker H, Measham F, Aldridge J (1995) Drug futures. Changing patterns of drug use amongst English youth. Institute for the Study of Drug Dependence, London
49. McC Miller P, Plant M (1996) Drinking, smoking, and illicit drug use among 15 and 16 year olds in the United Kingdom. British Medical Journal 313:394-397
50. Rudat K, Speed M, Ryan H (1992) Today's young adults: 16-19-year-olds look at alcohol, smoking, drugs and sexual behaviour. Health Education Authority, London
51. Rudnick G, Wall SC (1992) The molecular mechanism of "ecstasy" [3,4-methylenedioxymethamphetamine (MDMA)]: serotonin transporters are targets for MDMA induced serotonin release. Proc Nat Acad Sci 89:1817-1821
52. Fuller RW, Hines CW, Mills J (1965) Lowering of brain Serotonin level by Chloramphetamines. Biochem Pharmacol 14:483-488
53. Pletscher A, Burkard WP, Brunderer H, Grey KF (1963) Decrease of cerebral 5-hydroxytryptamine and 5-hydroxyindolacetic acid by an arylalkylamine. Life Sciences 2:828-833
54. Johnson MP, Hoffman AJ, Nichols DE (1986) Effects of the enantiomers of MDA, MDMA and related analogues on [^{3}H]serotonin and [^{3}H]dopamine release from the superfused rat brain slices. Eur J Pharmacol 132:269-276
55. Nichols DE, Lloyd DH, Hoffman AJ, Nichols MB, Yim GKW (1982) Effects of certain hallucinogenic amphetamine analogues on the release of (3H) Serotonin from rat brain synaptosomes. J Med Chem 25:535-538
56. Schmidt CJ, Levin JA, Lovenberg W (1987) In vitro and in vivo neurochemical effects of methylenedioxymethamphetamine on striatal monoaminergic systems in the rat brain. Biochem Pharmacol 36:747-755
57. Clineschmidt BV, Totaro JA, McGuffin JC, Pflueger AB (1976) Fenfluramine: long-term reduction in brain Serotonin (5-hydroxytryptamine). Eur J Pharmacol 35:211-214
58. Ricaurte G, Bryan G, Strauss L, Seiden L, Schuster C (1985) Hallucinogenic amphetamine selectively destroys brain serotonin terminals. Science 229:986-988
59. McKenna DJ, Peroutka SJ (1990) Neurochemistry and neurotoxicity of 3,4 methylenedioxymethamphetamine (MDMA, "ecstasy"). J Neurochem 54:14-22
60. Dowling GP, McDonagh ET III, Bost RO (1987) Eve and Ecstasy. A report of five deaths associated with the use of MDEA and MDMA. JAMA 257:1615-1617

61. Henry JA, Jeffreys KJ, Dawling S (1992) Toxicity and deaths from 3,4-methylene-dioxymethamphetamine (Ecstasy). Lancet 340:384-387
62. Screaton GR, Singer M, Cairns HS, Thrasher A, Sarner M, Cohen SL (1992) Hyperpyrexia and rhabdomyolysis after MDMA (ecstasy) abuse. Lancet 339:677-678.
63. Nimmo SM, Kennedy BW, Tullett WM, Blyth AS, Dougall JR (1993) Drug-induced hyperthermia. Anaesthesia 48:892-895
64. Singarajah C, Lavies NG (1992) An overdose of ecstasy. A role for dantrolene. Anaesthesia 47:686-687
65. Logan AS, Stickle B, O'Keefe N, Hewitson H (1993) Survival following ecstasy ingestion with a peak temperature of 42 degrees C. Anaesthesia 48:1017-1018
66. Webb C, Williams V (1993) Ecstasy intoxication: appreciation of complications and the role of dantrolene. Anaesthesia 48:542-543
67. Tehan B, Hardern R, Bodenham A (1993) Hyperthermia associated with 3,4-methyl-enedioxyethamphetamine (Eve). Anaesthesia 48:507-510
68. Rhodes PJ, Rhodes RS (1984) Elimination kinetics and symptomatology of diazepam withdrawal in abusers. Clin Toxicol 22:371
69. Marchant B, Wray R, Leach A, Nama M (1989) Flumazenil causing convulsions and ventricular tachycardia. Br Med J 299:860
70. Shulgin AT (1980) LSD. J Psychedelic Drugs 12:173
71. Khun DM, White FJ, Appel JB (1978) The discriminative stimulus properties of LSD: mechanisms of action. Neuropharmacology 17:257
72. McCarron MM, Schulze BW, Thompson GA (1981) Acute phencyclidine intoxication: clinical patterns, complications and treatment. Ann Emerg Med 10:290
73. Barton CH, Sterling ML, Vaziri ND (1981) Phencyclidine intoxication: clinical experience in 27 cases confirmed by urine assay. Ann Emerg Med 10:243

Chapter 16

Common PACU problems in trauma patients

W. Lingnau

Prehospital resuscitation and transportation to an emergency room for further diagnostic assessment and aggressive stabilisation of vital organ functions are cornerstones of the initial management of injured patients. The anaesthetist aims at circulatory stability and sufficient respiratory function. Surgical intervention to stop haemorrhage and to fix long bone fractures are at the top of the priority list for subsequent treatment in the operation room. Trauma patients are then referred to a Postanaesthesia Care Unit (PACU) or an Intensive Care Unit (ICU) depending on the severity of injury and the expected duration of impaired organ function. Tissue injury, hypoxaemia and haemorrhagic shock initiate pathophysiologic, immunologic and metabolic changes that lead to secondary complications. Wudel et al. [1] studied trauma patients after mass transfusion of more than 20 units and found 28% dying within the first 24 h and another 20% dying later from multiple organ failure. Patients who are specifically prone to complications are defined by advanced age, pretraumatic health condition, shock and the severity of injuries.

The PACU nurses and anaesthetists must be alert to recognise problems in these patients. By far the most frequent group of PACU problems relate to respiratory insufficiency, followed by postoperative hypothermia, cardiovascular and renal failure.

Respiratory failure

Respiratory failure is a frequent postinjury problem. All trauma patients can be expected to develop some degree of respiratory insufficiency. The coexistence of respiratory failure and trauma has been recognised since the early part of this century [2]. Today's PACU physicians should anticipate this clinical problem as a part of the lung's normal pathophysiologic response to tissue injury and shock. The incidence of respiratory problems increases with the number of present risk factors. A trivial injury may cause severe organ dysfunction in a vulnerable patient, for example, one with single or multiple rib fractures suffering from chronic obstructive lung disease (COPD). Long bone and pelvic fractures are known to cause adult respiratory distress syndrome mainly by immunologic activation. Finally, direct lung injury and chest contusion cause respiratory problems.

To understand the pathophysiology of respiratory failure one must split lung function into airway resistance and lung compliance, ventilation relative to matching perfused lung regions, diffusion and total surface area, and resulting work of breathing. Acute and trauma related respiratory dysfunction may add up to chronic lung disease. Advances in technology have led to the development of the Bicore monitor. This device determines intraoesophageal pressure to estimate intrapleural pressure. Muscle force is the product of pressure and frequency. Since the work of breathing is the product of respiratory muscle force and tidal volume, the Bicore monitor allows us to minimise the patients' cost of breathing during assisted ventilation. While breathing spontaneously, patients tend to adopt breathing patterns that minimise the work of breathing. The PACU anaesthetist may observe rapid shallow breaths in patients with stiff lungs and distinguish from large tidal volumes at slow rates in patients suffering from COPD.

Preexisting diseases

Chronic obstruction is best described by reduced forced expiratory volume in the first second and increased dead space (lung area that is ventilated but not perfused). Chronic hypoventilation in later stages causes increased arterial blood carbon dioxide and compensatory metabolic alkalosis. These patients are at a specific risk to develop lower respiratory tract infections as a consequence of impaired mucocilliary clearance. Further, a history of recurrent pulmonary infections mandates antibiotic prophylaxis that covers gram-positive and gram-negative microorganisms.

Fibrosis, silicosis and sarcoidosis are restrictive lung diseases. The common pathology is reduced total lung capacity, increased elastic recoil and reduced lung compliance, and pulmonary vascular hypertension. Hypoxaemia results from reduced surface area and reduced diffusion capacity. Superimposed traumatic insults, i.e., pulmonary oedema or atelectasis, may cause severe PACU problems.

Neuromuscular or skeletal abnormalities directly affect respiratory muscle force. Weak and inefficient respiratory muscles combine with decreased compliance or increased residual volume in kyphoscoliosis. Again, superimposed trauma may inevitably lead to the need of mechanical ventilation.

Trauma-related respiratory problems

Nonpulmonary causes of respiratory insufficiency are head injuries leading to unconsciousness and reduced ventilatory drive. These trauma patients are at increased risk of aspiration. Further, neurologic pulmonary oedema occurs secondary to massive sympathetic discharge mediated by the hypothalamus. It appears clinically as a fulminant pulmonary congestion and alveolar haemorrhage [3, 4]. Second, reduced cardiac performance due to cardiac contusion or cardiac tamponade causes congestion, stiffness, oedema, and reduced gas exchange. Subsequently, reduced organ perfusion leads to reduced mixed venous oxygen tension. In turn, reduced cerebral perfusion directs to reduced ventilatory drive. Third, musculoskeletal injuries, especially vertebral column injuries with associated spinal cord transection, have devastating effects on respiratory function, with long and difficult clinical courses.

Pulmonary contusion occurs frequently in blunt trauma [5]. The area of contusion is more susceptible to increased microvascular permeability. Clinical treatment should include "conservative" fluid resuscitation guided with pulmonary artery catheters. Crystalloids as well as colloids will leak into the injured area, hence, there is no proven advantage of one or the other. In areas of pulmonary contusion the cellular and humoral immunologic activation may lead to generalised acute lung injury [6]. Younger patients have more compliant thoracic cages. Therefore, they are more prone to the development of lung injury, but less to respiratory insufficiency after rib fractures. A specific problem is the development of a tension pneumothorax. Reduced venous return causes decreased cardiac output and, accordingly, reduced organ perfusion.

Atelectasis is a frequent PACU problem in traumatised patients. It describes a part of the lung that is not ventilated but at least partly perfused. The resulting effect is a loss of gas exchange in the affected lung region, and increased venous admixture. Atelectasis occurs as the result of collapse of an entire lung, lobe, or lung segment, or it can occur in a diffuse pattern. Bronchial obstruction from secretion or blood is a frequent cause of atelectasis. Deep one lung intubation at the site of an accident causes collapse of the opposite lung and is a serious complication. Pneumothorax occurs as a result of direct lung or airway injury from trauma, rib fractures, or attempts at percutaneous vascular cannulation. Pneumothorax causes hypoxaemia due to atelectasis and an intrapulmonary shunt. Treatment includes insertion of a chest tube for drainage, bronchoscopy and bronchial toilet, sitting in an upright position and early mobilisation. Continuous positive airway pressure (CPAP) and incentive spirometry are cornerstones of respiratory therapy.

Arterial hypoxaemia may be present in posttraumatic patients who have no discernible change in the chest radiograph. Perhaps these patients have an increased right-to-left intrapulmonary shunt due to diffuse airway collapse. The relationship between the functional residual capacity (FRC) of the lung and closing capacity is a prime determinant of this effect [7, 8]. Any situation that results in either an increased closing capacity, i.e., increasing age, or reduced FRC (pulmonary oedema, infection, aspiration, obesity) will place the patient at increased risk of hypoxaemia.

Pulmonary oedema is another process that can result in hypoxaemia in the postoperative period. Cooperman and Price examined 40 cases of perioperative pulmonary oedema and found one-half the patients to have preoperative evidence of cardiovascular disease. The most common time of appearance of pulmonary oedema was observed within 60 min of completion of surgery [9]. More than one half these cases were preceded by hypertension, suggesting that this problem may be related to the high pulmonary vascular pressures seen in acute postoperative hypertension.

Fat embolisation syndrome and mediators of lung injury

Fat embolism occurs with any major fracture, typically with long bone and pelvic fractures. Key symptoms are acute lung injury, mental status changes, thrombocytopenia, and petechial rash on the chest. There are three major hypotheses of the aetiology. Causative factors may include the extrusion of intramedullary fat tissue into circulation [10, 11], aggregation of circulating chylomicrons into fat droplets [12], or damage from free fatty acids liberated by lipases [13]. Clinical signs are hypoxaemia and increased dead space. Patients develop pulmonary oedema because of a high hydrostatic pressure in the pulmonary capillaries, an increased capillary permeability, or following sustained reductions in the interstitial hydrostatic pressure. The latter type of pulmonary oedema is seen following prolonged airway obstruction. [14, 15]. In patients with a permeability injury, pulmonary oedema can be exacerbated by increases in hydrostatic pressure. Pulmonary oedema characterised by a permeability injury is seen following disseminated intravascular coagulation (DIC), shock, trauma, massive transfusion, sepsis, and anaphylaxis. This type of pulmonary oedema is frequently called the adult respiratory distress syndrome (ARDS), and is characterised by hypoxaemia, diffuse pulmonary infiltrates on radiographs, and reduced lung compliance. A common early pathologic finding is neutrophil accumulation in the lung vasculature and tissue. There is increasing evidence that activation of arachidonic acid metabolites, the prostaglandins and the leukotrienes, may be responsible for the permeability injury seen in humans [16]. Experimentally, leukotriene D4 increases pulmonary permeability. [17]. While modern management of orthopaedic injuries (early stabilisation [18]) has markedly reduced the incidence of fat emboli syndrome, steroids have no benefit in established acute lung injury [19].

Hypothermia

Hypothermia prolongs the recovery room stay [20]. Drug metabolism is markedly decreased by perioperative hypothermia. The duration of action of vecuronium is more than doubled by 2°C of core hypothermia. Coagulation is impaired by mild hypothermia. The most important factor appears to be a cold-induced defect in platelet function. Hypothermia can contribute to wound infections both by directly impairing immune function [21] and by triggering thermoregulatory vasoconstriction that in turn decreases wound oxygen delivery [22]. Profound hypothermia (<33°C), finally, can produce unconsciousness.

The major adverse effects are patient discomfort, vasoconstriction, and shivering. Shivering increases metabolic rate and hence the need to increase cardiac output and minute ventilation. Not all patients who shiver postoperatively are hypothermic, suggesting that the mechanism of this event may be related to inadequate descending control of spinal reflexes following inhalation anaesthesia. Shivering occurs in patients who have lost body heat during the surgical procedure or as a neurological effect of volatile anaesthetic agents [23, 24]. Shivering is to be avoided, either by warming the patient in the operating room or by giving small doses of tranquilising drugs. In the PACU, hypothermic patients should have supplemental oxygen, warm intravenous fluids and blood, and external warming. External warming can be accomplished with thermal blankets or thermal ceilings, which lower oxygen consumption.

Cardiovascular problems

Cardiovascular complications are, in order of decreasing frequency, hypotension, arrhythmias, hypertension, and myocardial infarction. History of heart failure or coronary artery disease complicate PACU treatment. Postoperative vasodilatation is caused by increasing temperature either during rewarming or as a consequence of systemic inflammation. Coronary perfusion may further deteriorate with reduced diastolic arterial pressures. Treatment with dopamine (4-10 µg/kg/per min), norepinephrine or dobutamine support cardiovascular function. Agitation, hypertension, and arrhythmias are likely to occur in the patient who is having pain or is being stimulated by the presence of an endotracheal tube and has too little analgesia or sedation. Hypotension often accompanies respiratory depression in the patient who is sedated but not stimulated. Pain treatment should be anticipated and begun before the patient emerges from anaesthesia in order to avoid agitation and sympathetic stimulation in the immediate postanaesthetic period. Regional anaesthetic techniques, i.e., thoracic epidural anaesthesia or intercostal blockades after rib fractures, not only improve respiratory function but also help to maintain cardiac performance.

Renal failure

Posttraumatic renal failure may either develop early after injury secondary to hypotension or inadequate resuscitation, or days to weeks later for a variety of reasons. Again, preexisting diseases predispose for additional PACU complications. The elderly trauma patient in particular may reach the emergency department with creatinine levels within the upper reference limits. In light of reduced muscle mass, this represents elevated values, and creatinine clearances are below 50 ml/min. Nonoliguric renal failure is the most common form of renal dysfunction [25-28]. Shin et al. [29] found the incidence of posttraumatic renal failure to decrease steadily, but nonoliguric renal dysfunction increased from 10% to 73% during the 5-year observation period [29]. About 2% of severely injured patients require extracorporeal renal replacement therapy, of which 35% are due to inadequate resuscitation and 65% as a part of multiple organ failure syndrome.

Causes of posttraumatic renal failure are haemorrhagic or cardiogenic shock (cardiac tamponade, tension pneumothorax), increased abdominal pressure (retroperitoneal haematoma following pelvic fracture), haemoglobinuria or myoglobinuria (crush injury, mass transfusion, electrical injuries), drugs (radiocontrast agents) or sepsis. Most often, renal dysfunction is not the result of one insult but of either recurrent events or a combination of insults. Anuria may be a obstructive problem subsequent to urethral or ureteral injury, urinary blood clots or retroperitoneal haematoma. Back-leakage of up to 50% of glomerular filtration rate (GFR) into the renal interstitium may then cause an interstitial oedema.

Recovery from morphine-based anaesthetics or neuromuscular blockade is often a function of the dose and agent administered and of postoperative renal function.

Kidneys receive 25% of cardiac output, and autoregulation maintains renal blood flow constant between mean arterial pressures of 75 and 160 mm Hg. Renal arterial wall tension sets renal arterial tone by intrinsic myogenic reflexes. However, both reduced renal blood flow in response to afferent vasoconstriction and efferent vasodilatation decrease the GFR. The glomerular filtration fraction (120 ml/min) is 20% of renal blood flow. The renal medulla is hypoxic (PaO_2=10 mm Hg) under normal conditions and hence is particularly sensitive to reduced peritubular capillary blood flow. In contrast, tubules demonstrate the highest metabolic needs to perform active reabsorption of sodium. There is evidence that reduction of transport activity, as with furosemide, relieves medullar hypoxia [30]. Conversely, mannitol and acetazolamide aggravate medullar hypoxia, while medullar blood flow remains a fundamental determinant of regional oxygen tension. There are clinical studies [31-33] as well as anecdotal experience that high dose furosemide improves urine flow and may prevent oliguria in conjunction with dopamine. However, furosemide-induced forced diuresis appears to provide no measurable benefit with respect to mortality and length of stay [31]. Furosemide should be ineffective in oliguric patients. It acts on the luminal side of the ascending tubules and hence can only work if there is sufficient glomerular filtration. In combination with aminoglycosides or vancomycin, furosemide induces or enhances renal- and ototoxicity.

Conclusions and clinical implications

The posttraumatic patient in the PACU is subject to respiratory, thermoregulatory, cardiovascular and renal complications. Organ function should therefore be monitored carefully. Vigorous volume repletion after haemorrhage is the first prerequisite of preventive measures. Treatment of hypoxaemia by face-mask oxygen is effective in restoring the PaO_2 in many cases. If hypoxaemia persists (PaO_2<60 mm Hg) despite maximal oxygen therapy (FIO_2 1.0), tracheal intubation and mechanical ventilation should be initiated. In such patients ventilation with PEEP will increase the functional residual capacity and result in an improvement in arterial oxygenation. Continuous positive airway pressure by an external mask (mask or nasal CPAP) is used for treatment of patients with severe hypoxaemia who have adequate carbon dioxide elimination. Incentive spirometry and bronchial toilet are mandatory. Regional anaesthesia has been used for the relief of postoperative pain to avoid narcotic-induced respiratory depression. Hypothermia causes shivering and elevated oxygen consumption and hence should be reversed as early as possible. Cardiovascular treatment includes dopamine (2.5-4-10 µg/kg/per min), dobutamine or phenylephrine after adequate volume resuscitation. Renal failure is best prevented by maintained organ perfusion as a consequence of normovolaemia and normotension. The target of urine flow is at least 0.5 ml/kg/per hour. Patients are discharged to the ward in stable haemodynamic conditions after arterial blood gas analysis and adequate pain management. Transfer is confirmed and signed by the PACU physician.

References

1. Wudel JH, Morris JA Jr, Yates K, Wilson A, Bass SM (1991) Massive transfusion: outcome in blunt trauma patients. J Trauma 31:1-7
2. Brewer LA, Burbank B, Samson PC et al (1946) The wet lung in war casualities. Ann Surg 123:343-347
3. Graf CJ, Rossi NP (1978) Catecholamine response to intracranial hypertension. J Neurosurg 49:862-868
4. Moss J, Lisbon A, Levine JF (1975) The effects of increased intracranial pressure on respiratory functions. In: Lundberg N, Ponten U, Brock M (eds) Intracranial pressure II. Springer-Verlag, Berlin Heidelberg New York, p 315
5. Wagner RB, Jamieson PM (1989) Pulmonary contusion. Evaluation and classification by computed tomography. Surg Clin North Am 69:31-40
6. Pepe PE, Potkin RT, Reus DH, Hudson LD, Carrico CJ (1982) Clinical predictors of the adult respiratory distress syndrome. Am J Surg 144:124-130
7. Hamilton WK (1961) Atelectasis, pneumothorax, and aspiration as postoperative complications. Anesthesiology 22:708-713
8. Don HF, Wahba WM, Craig DB (1972) Airway closure, gas trapping, and the functional residual capacity during anesthesia. Anesthesiology 36:533-539
9. Cooperman LH, Price HR (1970) Pulmonary edema in the operative and postoperative period: review of 40 cases. Ann Surg 172:883-891
10. Morton KS, Kendall MJ (1965) Fat embolism: its production and source of fat. Can J Surg 8:214
11. Peltiere LF (1956) Fat embolism III. The toxic properties of neutral fat and free fatty acids. Surgery 40:665
12. Lequire VS, Shapiro JL, Lequire CB et al (1959) A study of the pathogenesis of fat embolism based on human necropsy material and animal experiments. Am J Pathol 35:999
13. Moylan JA, Birnbaum M, Katz A, Everson MA (1976) Fat emboli syndrome. J Trauma 16:341-347
14. Weissman C, Damask MC, Yang J (1984) Noncardiogenic pulmonary edema following laryngeal obstruction. Anesthesiology 60:163-165
15. Jackson FN, Rowland V, Corssen G (1980) Laryngospasm induced pulmonary edema. Chest 78:819-821
16. Crandall ED, Staub NE, Goldberg HS, Effros RM (1983) Recent development in pulmonary edema. Ann Intern Med 99:808-822
17. Shapiro JM, Mihm FG, Trudell JR, Stevens JH, Feeley TW (1987) Leukotriene D4 increases extravascular lung water in the dog. Circ Shock 21:121-128
18. Goris RJ, Gimbrere JS, van Niekerk JL, Schoots FJ, Booy LH (1982) Early osteosynthesis and prophylactic mechanical ventilation in the multitrauma patient. J Trauma 22:895-903
19. Bernard GR, Luce JM, Sprung CL, Rinaldo JE, Tate RM, Sibbald WJ, Kariman K, Higgins S, Bradley R, Metz CA et al (1987) High-dose corticosteroids in patients with the adult respiratory distress syndrome. N Engl J Med 317:1565-1570
20. Hines R, Barash PG, Watrous G, O'Connor T (1992) Complications occurring in the postanaesthesia care unit: a survey. Anesth Analg 74:503-509
21. Van Oss CJ, Absolom DR, Moore LL, Park-BH, Humbert-JR (1980) Effect of temperature on the chemotaxis, phagocytic engulfment, digestion and O2 consumption of human polymorphonuclear leukocytes. J Reticuloendothel Soc 27:561-564

22. Sheffield CW, Hopf HW, Sessler DI (1993) Local heat reverses the decrease in subcutaneous oxygen tension produced by thermoregulatory vasoconstriction. Anesth Analg 76:S389
23. Sessler DI, Olofsson CI, Rubinstein EH (1988) The thermoregulatory threshold in humans during nitrous oxide-fentanyl anesthesia. Anesthesiology 69:357-364
24. Sessler DI, Israel D, Pozos RS, Pozos M, Rubinstein EH (1988) Spontaneous post-anesthetic tremor does not resemble thermoregulatory shivering. Anesthesiology 68:843-850
25. Myers BD, Miller DC, Mehigan JT, Olcott CO, Golbetz H, Robertson CR, Derby G, Spencer R, Friedman S (1984) Nature of the renal injury following total renal ischemia in man. J Clin Invest 73:329-341
26. Lordon RE, Burton JR (1972) Posttraumatic renal failure in military personnel in Southeast Asia. Am J Med 53:137-147
27. Anderson RJ, Linas SL, Berns AS, Henrich WL, Miller-TR, Gabow-PA, Schrier-RW (1977) Nonoliguric acute renal failure. N Engl J Med 296:1134-1138
28. Dixon BS, Anderson RJ (1985) Nonoliguric acute renal failure. Am J Kidney Dis 6:71-80
29. Shin B, Mackenzie CF, Cowley RA (1979) Changing pattern of posttraumatic acute renal failure. Am Surg 45:182-189
30. Brezis M, Agmon Y, Epstein FH (1994) Determinants of intrarenal oxygenation. Am J Physiol 267:F1059-F1062
31. Brown CB, Ogg CS, Cameron JS (1981) High dose furosemide in acute renal failure: a controlled trial. Clin Nephrol 15:90-96
32. Graziani G, Cantaluppi A, Casati S, Citterio A, Scalamogna A, Aroldi A, Silenzio R, Brancaccio D, Ponticelli C (1984) Dopamine and furosemide in oliguric acute renal failure. Nephron 37:39-42
33. Parker S, Graziano CC, Isaac M, Howland WS, Kahn RC (1981) Dopamine administration in oliguria and oliguric renal failure. Crit Care Med 9:630-632

Chapter 17

Three-in-one block as locoregional analgesia for hip fractures

K. Bronselaer, M. Gillis, H. Delooz

The three-in-one block (3 in 1) of the lower limb is a technique for blocking the femoral, lateral cutaneous femoris and obturator nerve as first described by Winnie et al. in 1973 [1]. On an anatomical and theoretical background Winnie proposed in the original article a technique using a similar concept as the one that applies to the brachial plexus block.

He hypothesized that a similar nerve sheath was formed by the fascia of the abdominal muscles around the femoral nerve so that the injection of a sufficient amount (20-40 ml) of a local anaesthetic would spread cephalic until it reaches the lumbar plexus and then blocks the roots at the lumbar level L 2 to L 4. These roots are the origin of the femoral, lateral cutaneous femoris and obturator nerve.

Although cadaver studies could not show such a sheath, the injection of a sufficient amount of local anaesthetic by the technique described produces a sensory block to the three nerves sufficient to provide analgesia and even anaesthesia of the upper, lateral part of the leg [2]. The cadaver studies also showed that when using an amount of 40 ml of colored dye, both the femoral and the lateral cutaneous femoris nerve were stained and, thus, when using this amount of local anaesthetic, both nerves would be blocked as well [2]. Winnie et al. and Seeberger et al. even demonstrated that the injection of 40 ml of local anaesthetic probably also blocks at least the sensory fibers of the obturator nerve [1-3].

Within the next decades the incidence of hip fracture will increase from 1.46 million in 1990 to 6.26 millions in 2050. The population at risk is also an elderly population so all these people presenting at the emergency department should be able to profit from an easy to perform, time-saving and inexpensive technique, without any risk of side effects caused by the use of general analgesic techniques [4-6].

Technique

An indwelling intravenous cannula is placed and intravenous perfusion is started. The patient's blood pressure, heart rhythm, heart frequency and oxygen saturation are monitored.

The lumbar plexus is enclosed within a sheath of connective tissue which can be entered at the level of the inguinal ligament, where the femoral nerve enters the thigh. Local anaesthetic injected at this point will spread cephalic in this perineural sheath between the iliacus and the psoas muscles. A blockade of all the branches of the lumbar plexus is created when enough volume of local anaesthetic is used. The technique used according to Bruce Scott [7] anaesthetizes the femoral, obturator and the lateral cutaneous nerve of the thigh, which gives an easy and excellent analgesia without major complications.

For this technique, there are two sets of needles commercially available. The single shot set consists of a fully insulated needle with an injection side port. The catheter set consists of the same insulated needle with a cannula that can be placed into the femoral nerve sheath following the injection of the full dose of local anaesthetic. Through this cannula a small catheter is placed for continuous infusion of local anaesthetic.

The patient lies in supine position. After shaving the inguinal region, the skin is disinfected with a non-alcohol-containing disinfectant. After placing a large sterile compress on the pubis, the patient is covered with sterile blankets in such a manner that the upper thigh and the patella are still visible.

The identification of the femoral pulse is carried out where the pulse is easiest to palpate. This can be at the level of the inguinal ligament or somewhat lower. At 1-1.5 cm lateral to the artery only a tiny amount of local anaesthetic is given subcutaneously before the skin is punctured with a stylet. With the index finger still on the pulse of the femoral artery, the needle is inserted. This needle is connected to a nerve stimulator. This electrical nerve stimulator is used to elicit small and painless muscle twitches in order to give correct information about the localization of the nerve.

The needle is advanced slowly cephalic at about 60° from the skin until the nerve stimulator causes movement of the vastus medianus muscle and the patella.

The intensity of the pulses is started at 0.6 mA and increased if necessary until twitches are seen. Then an attempt is made to lower the electric pulses by steps of 0.2 mA until just a hint of a twitch can be seen. While the anaesthetist is keeping the needle strictly immobile, 2 ml of the mixture of local anaesthetic are injected following aspiration by an assistant. This injection should make the twitches disappear. Then – using the single-shot technique – a total of 40 ml of a mixture of local anaesthetic is injected while aspiration is performed after every 10 ml.

If the catheter technique is used, the cannula is advanced in the perineural space after injecting 35 ml of local anaesthetic with intermittent aspiration. The catheter is placed through the cannula with a slight resistance at the tip and for about 10 cm in the perineural space. A bacterial filter is attached at the end of the catheter; the remaining 5 ml is used to flush the catheter and filter this catheter is sutured to the skin. A water-resistant, transparent dressing covers the puncture side.

The total amount of local anaesthetic should be lowered for patients with heart disease (NYHA class 3 and 4) [8].

When the catheter technique is used the patients can, furthermore, receive an infusion of 15 mg/h bupivacaine 0.25%.

Study

Aim, technique and study population

As there are no studies with this technique in an emergency department known to us, we conducted a double-blind study with three mixtures of local anaesthetics. We used the catheter technique as described. We also evaluated this technique as a means to provide an easy, safe and comfortable way of pain relief for fractures of the femur head and the upper third of the femoral shaft. We used the Linear Visual Analog Score (LVAS) to study the analgesic effects. Sixty-one consecutive patients presenting with a hip fracture at our emergency department were evaluated.

Results

As shown in Figure 1, the LVAS declined from 8-9 to 2-4 at 5 min, and to 1-2 at 15 min after injection of the local anaesthetics. We could not demonstrate a statistically significant difference between the three groups in time of onset or in analgesic effect.

Complications and side effects

Three of our patients showed toxic side effects of the local anaesthetics. Two of them presented nonmalignant cardiac dysrhythmia and one complained of numbness of the tongue, dizziness and double vision. All of these side effects subsided within 10 min without treatment.

We had only four failures of the bloc due to technical reasons. In two patients we could not locate the pulse of the femoral artery due to obesity or a local hematoma

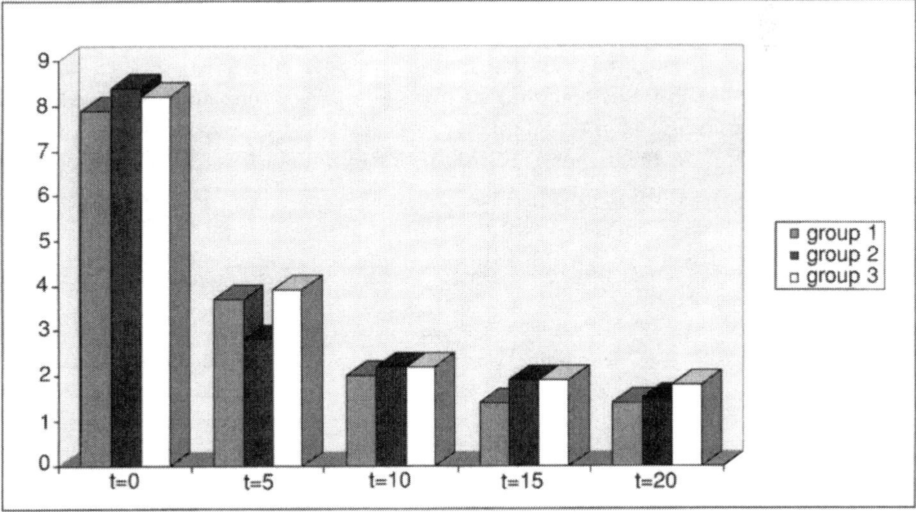

Fig. 1. Evolution of the LVAS in time for the three groups

and we were not able to stimulate the femoral nerve. In one patient we used too much local anaesthetic before puncturing the skin and we were not able to stimulate the femoral nerve. In the last one we aspirated blood after injecting the first 5 ml of local anaesthetic mixture after which stimulation to redirect the needle was no longer possible.

Discussion

As shown in Figure 1, this technique provides a very good analgesic effect in a very short time. The side effects are few and easy avoidable. The most common complications are primarily due to the rather high amount of local anaesthetic needed to block all three nerves in elderly people with low body weight.

The nature of the toxic side effects of local anaesthetics are divided into systemic and local toxicity. The systemic toxicity involves the central nervous system (CNS) and cardiovascular system. The initial symptoms of CNS local anaesthetic toxicity consist of a generalized feeling of light-headedness, dizziness, auditory and visual disturbances and tinnitus. Drowsiness, disorientation and a temporary lack of consciousness may also occur. Cardiovascular toxicity such as dysrhythmia, depression of myocardial contractility and peripheral vasodilatation occur more frequently with direct intravascular injection [9]. Indeed, since this technique requires an injection up to 40 ml of local anaesthetic near the femoral artery, an intravascular injection or a high absorption into the bloodstream can easily occur.

Local irritation of the nerve with a transient burning sensation is caused by the injection in close contact with the nerve. Puncture of the femoral artery can result in a local hematoma which normally subsides in a few days.

Conclusions

Both the single-shot and the catheter technique of the 3 in 1 block are easy to perform and only require a few skills which are easy to learn and very well feasible in the emergency setting. Both techniques give an excellent analgesia with none or minimal manipulation of the patient. When using local anaesthetics with a long duration of action or the catheter technique, the same block can be used for perioperative and even postoperative analgesia with minimal side effects.

References

1. Winnie AP et al (1973) The inguinal perivascular technique of lumbar plexus anaesthesia, the "three in one" block. Anaesth Analg 52:989-996
2. Ritter JW (1995) Femoral nerve "sheath" for inguinal paravascular lumbar plexus block is not found in human cadavers. J Clin Anaesth 7:470-473
3. Seeberger MD, Urwyler A (1995) Paravascular lumbar plexus block: block extension after femoral nerve stimulation and injection of 20 vs 40 ml mepivacaine 10 mg/ml. Acta Anaesthesiol Scand 39:769-773

4. Johnell O (1997) The socioeconomic burden of fractures: today and in the 21st century. Am J Med 103:20s-25s
5. Lauritzen JB (1997) Hip fractures. Epidemiology, risk factors, falls, energy absorption, hip protectors and prevention. Dan Med Bull 44:155-168
6. Kannus P et al (1996) Epidemiology of hip fractures. Bone 18:57s-63s
7. Scott DB (1989) Techniques of regional anaesthesia. Medi Globe, Switzerland, pp 122-123
8. Criteria Committee, New York Heart Association (1964) Diseases of the heart and blood vessels; nomenclature and criteria for diagnosis, 6th edn. Little and Brown, Boston, p 114
9. Concepcion M, Covino BG (1984) Rational use of local anaesthetics. Drugs 27:256-270

Chapter 18

Recommendations for blood transfusion in trauma patients

F. Mercuriali, G. Inghilleri

Trauma is a major health care problem, with an impact on every hospital and blood bank. Despite relevant improvement in the management of trauma victims, blunt or penetrating injuries from different causes are the leading cause of death for subjects under 40 in developed countries and they continue to exert a major impact on blood resources worldwide.

Although the majority of trauma patient are managed without blood transfusion those who need transfusion support may require large amounts of blood components, in some cases in emergency situations. Thus correct strategies for transfusion therapy in trauma patients may have important implications for blood bank inventory. Moreover, beside the impact on inventory, appropriate transfusion practice is of critical relevance for the patient's clinical outcome. As with any medicinal product, blood and blood products can be of great benefit to the patient if used properly, but incorrect use can cause harm. Among the well recognised complications of blood transfusion (transmission of infectious disease, immunologic reactions and immunomodulation), in the setting of trauma patients there is a need for special concern regarding the risk of acute hemolytic reactions and alterations in immune functions.

The problem of acute hemolytic reactions usually due to clerical error will be discussed below. The clinical importance of immunomodulatory effects of allogeneic blood transfusion has been the topic of a number of studies in surgical patients [1-6]. Although controversies still exist, in most reports transfusion was found to be a predictor of postoperative infection. As trauma patients, especially those with shock, become immune compromised and are at high risk for infections and multiple organ failure, the adoption of prudent strategies for allogeneic blood transfusion and the appropriate use of its alternatives seems to be advisable in this setting.

Unfortunately no specific transfusion guidelines address the problem of transfusion therapy in trauma patients. However some indications can be derived from the general transfusion guidelines published by different scientific associations [7-14], from guidelines on global management of trauma patients [15-16] and by few studies involving particular groups of trauma patients.

As far as transfusion practice is concerned, beside those who can be managed without blood transfusion, trauma patients can be subdivided into three main categories:
1. patients who are treated for many days in the intensive care unit (ICU) because of the traumatic event;

2. patients expected to suffer an acute and consistent blood loss and shock requiring large volumes of blood;
3. patients in whom consistent transfusion support is predicted over the entire hospital stay, mainly as a consequence of surgery (semi-urgent patients).

Patients in the ICU

Anemia is common in ICU patients and results in the frequent use of RBC transfusions. Out of 4875 consecutive patients admitted to six Canadian tertiary level intensive care units, 28% received erythrocyte transfusions [17]. The most frequent reasons for anemia, and subsequent blood transfusion, are acute bleeding (35%) and the augmentation of O_2 delivery (25%). However one of the major reasons for anemia is blood loss associated with frequent and multiple phlebotomies for laboratory monitoring. It has been estimated that patients in the ICU receive three to five phlebotomies per day with a mean volume of blood withdrawn during the ICU stay of approximately 1 l [18]. Moreover it has been recently demonstrated that the erythropoietin (EPO) response to anemia is severly blunted in critically ill patients. Thus inadequate EPO production is likely to contribute to the development of anemia in these patients [19].

In critically ill patients an optimal and safe transfusion trigger has not been defined, as several studies have suggested that relatively high values of hematocrit, augmenting O_2 delivery, may decrease mortality while others claimed that the immunomodulatory effect and the microcirculatory alterations [20] induced by RBC transfusion may be detrimental.

In the literature there is great variation in reported transfusion practice both in the perioperative period and in critical care [21, 22]. In the majority of studies no significant difference between groups maintained on different transfusion regimens, and consequently at different Hb values, was observed, as far as mortality rates, development of organ dysfunction or failure, length of stay in ICU, hospital stay or intervention rates were concerned.

Two studies [23, 24] have documented increased mortality rates in patients who exhibited pathologic O_2 supply dependency, which can be an indication of tissue hypoxia (responsible for multiple system organ failure followed by death). This suggested that O_2 delivery should be increased or maintained at a high level by increasing Hb levels through a liberal transfusion regimen, because in such circumstances the use of restrictive transfusion strategies would result in increased organ dysfunction and mortality rates. Several investigators advocated the need for maintaining high Hb levels in critically ill patients [25-28]. In high risk perioperative patients an hematocrit value of 33% (Hb 110 g/l) was recommended as part of resuscitation protocols [28].

However several studies have also been published in which it is noted that severe anemia in high risk surgical patients is well tolerated. In patients refusing allogeneic blood transfusion and in regions with limited blood supplies, anemia patients with Hb values below 5 g/l has not been correlated with higher mortality rates [29-32].

The contradictory results of published data prompted the development of randomized clinical trials comparing restrictive transfusion policies, aimed at maintaining Hb values between 70 and 90 g/l, with more liberal transfusion regimens, taking into consideration not only mortality rates (in ICU, during hospital stay and at 30 days) and survival times but also the assessment of organ dysfunction and multiple organ failure. Recently a multicenter prospective randomized study [33] was carried out in 69 normovolemic critically ill patients (including trauma patients) with Hb values below 90 g/l. Patients were randomized to receive RBC transfusions to maintain Hb values between 100 and 120 g/l or to maintain levels between 70 and 90 g/l. The two groups received a mean of 4.8 RBC units and 2.5 RBC units, respectively, per patient. The 30-day, 120-day and in-ICU mortality survival analysis and organ dysfunction scores were similar in the two groups.

Another study [34] of critically ill patients with sepsis evaluated the importance of maintaining an O_2 delivery >600 ml/min/m^2, adopting different strategies (fluid boluses, administration of blood products and the use of inotropes), compared to a standard therapy to obtain an O_2 delivery of 50-550 ml/min/m^2. Both groups of patients had the same incidence of complications, number of days in ventilation and intensive care and in hospital; however, patients who achieved O_2 delivery >600 ml/min/m^2 had significantly lower mortality (14%) than with patients with lower O_2 delivery (56%).

A review of the literature on this subject seems to indicate that Hb values between 70 and 90 g/l can be maintained in low-risk cardiac and noncardiac surgical patients. The randomized clinical trials did not demonstrate a difference in mortality and other parameters in critically ill patients maintained in the range of 70-90 g/l Hb compared with patients maintained with higher Hb values. However the number of patients in all these studies is too small to draw treatment guidelines suggesting the best transfusion policy in critically ill patients.

Recently, the potential role of recombinant human EPO has been evaluated in critically ill patients and found effective in reducing blood transfusion utilization in this setting [35].

Patients with hemorraghic shock

Hemorraghic shock after trauma is an emergency situation that may expose the patient to the risk of death. Shocked patients are subjected to two different types of risks: those connected with hemorrhage and shock and those related to the transfusion of very large amounts of stored blood.

During storage, blood suffers progressive loss of function and undergoes several metabolic and structural changes, termed "storage lesions" [36, 37]. These include: hemolysis, alteration of RBC deformability, microaggregate formation, release of vasoactive substances, increase of K-phosphate and ammonia, pH decrease, altered affinity of Hb for O_2, decrease of 2-3 DPG (diphosphoglycerate), reduction of intracellular ATP, denaturation of proteins (including coagulation factors) and platelet degeneration. Consequently the administration of large volume of stored blood may be responsible for relevant changes in the metabolic state of the patient.

However the depth and duration of shock represent more significant determinants of physiologic derangement than the transfusion of blood. Consequently the basic rule in the treatment of these patients is to give adequate fluid resuscitation (to assure an adequate volemia and organ perfusion) and RBCs (to maintain O_2 delivery), rather than adopting a conservative RBCs transfusion policy in order to avoid immediate or delayed transfusion risks [38]. Furthermore, normovolemia is a critical factor in maintaining hemostasis as hypovolemia leads to progressive acidosis which has been shown to enhance the appearance of hemostatic disturbances [39].

In these patients transfusion of a relevant volume of blood is a life saving procedure and has a very favourable risk to benefit ratio. Unfortunately it is difficult in these cases to suggest uniform guidelines because of a relative lack in the literature of detailed rigorous studies.

However an understanding of the pathophysiology and treatment of shock, a knowledge of appropriate indications for component therapy and familiarity with risks and alternatives could represent the basis for the development of strategies to optimally use blood components in this critical pathology, keeping in mind that the primary goal in patients with hemorrhagic shock is: 1) prompt restoration of the volemia in order to guarantee organ perfusion and subsequently provide O_2 flow to the cells; and 2) to adopt all the measures necessary to avoid further blood loss.

The clinical hallmarks of hemorragic shock are reduction of circulating volume, acidosis, hypothermia and frequently coagulopathy.

Reduction of circulating volume

During the course of hemorrhage the patient loses fluids and O_2 carrying capacity; moreover experimental work [38] has indicated that in the course of hemorrhagic shock extracellular fluids shift into the intracellular space due to the impairment of the energy dependent Na^+/K^+-ATP pump [40]. In these experiments it was also demonstrated that when only the shed blood was reinfused the survival of the animals was 20%, when 10 ml/kg of plasma was added, the survival improved to 30% and when lactate Ringers's was added to the shed blood 70% of the animals survived. This means that in hemorrhagic shock the most important measure is to restore volemia as hypoxia can be tolerated for considerable periods of time in most tissues.

Hypothermia

Shock is associated with loss of thermal regulation and decreased heat production [41]. However in shocked patients hypothermia develops mainly as a consequence of rapid infusions of large volumes of blood, components and resuscitation fluids and it is the most frequent and significant side effect of massive transfusion. Hypothermia induces an increased affinity of Hb for O_2, decreased platelet and coagulation factor function (also with normal levels of coagulation factors and number of platelets) and hypocalcemia (liver does not metabolize citrate).

Moreover when cold blood is rapidly infused through a central line with its tip near the sinoatrial node it can cause local hypothermia and a local decrease in ionized calcium, resulting in fatal arrythmias.

Hypothermia can be prevented or ameliorated by warming intravenous fluids and blood before infusion. The adoption of devices specifically indicated for blood warming is particularly important in order to avoid temperatures exceeding 40°C, because, in this case, shortened survival of RBCs or acute hemolysis may result.

Acidosis

If the hypoxia continues the energy demands (ATP production) are sustained by anaerobic conversion of glucose to lactate, which leads to the intracellular accumulation of hydrogen ions. The release from the cells of lactate and H+ ions produces acidosis that, together with the increased lactate levels and base deficit, is thought to be responsible for decreased cardiac contractility and increased mortality [42, 43]. However it has been demonstrated that a reduction of pH to values below 7 can be tolerated if hypoxia is promptly corrected. For this reason, concurrent with correction of volemia the O_2 carrying capacity should be restored through the transfusion of RBCs. Although stored blood has a low pH (mean 6.3), after massive transfusion the sodium citrate present in the anticoagulant is converted into sodium bicabonate in the liver and alkalosis usually occurs. Theoretically this could be detrimental because initially alkalosis increases Hb affinity for O_2; that, together with the progressive reduction of RBC 2-3-DPG occurring during storage, could decrease O_2 off-loading and consequently exacerbate hypoxia. Fortunately alkalosis stimulates enzymatic activity in the Embden-Meyerhof pathway of glycolysis, increasing intracellular 2-3-DPG with a consequent rapid restoration of O_2 unloading. Patients with adequate cardiac reserve can compensate, through increased cardiac output, the temporary hypoxia due to decreased O_2 unloading, but patients with poor cardiac reserve may be exposed to increased risks althrough the real clinical importance of this situation is not clear.

In patients with shock, the persistence of acidosis provides a marker for the need of additional resuscitation and not for the administration of bicarbonate. This should be avoided because: 1) it provides only a transient improvement of acidosis but may obscure the underlying tissue perfusion deficit; 2) it may result in more severe alkalosis with the undesierable effects of decreased myocardial contractility and increased affinity of Hb for O_2.

In the course of massive transfusion pH may range from 7.48 to 7.50 and it is usually associated with increased K^+ excretion, but during storage of blood, potassium concentration accumulates to reach values of 30-40 mEq/l after 3 weeks so that the transfusion of high volumes of stored blood might be responsible for hyperkalemia; however, with infusion of 100-150 ml/min of blood significant K^+ abnormalities rarely occur.

Many multitransfused patients with shock, unless renal function ceases, are hypokalemic because generally these patients have increased levels of aldosterone, antidiuretic and steroid hormones. In 471 patients receiving massive transfusion

47% had high and 18% low serum K^+ levels, but only 5% of them were hyperkalemic, once the acidosis was corrected. Hyperkalemia can be suspected by the modification of the ECG (elevated peak of T waves).

Transfusion practice in hemorraghic shock

The most frequently utilized guidelines for resuscitation of patients with hemorragic shock are those developed by the American College of Surgeon Committee on Trauma [15, 16]. These general guidelines allow an evaluation of the depth of shock and definition of the most appropriate means of fluid resuscitation based on the clinical symptoms of the presenting patients (Table 1).

Until control over the hemorrhage is gained, relaying on the hemoglobin concentration and the hematocrit measurements to determine adequate fluid and blood administration can be misleading. The appropriateness of therapy or the need for further fluid or blood support should be monitored by hemodynamic response and return of tissue perfusion (measured by mental status, urine output, capillary refill and absence of acidosis).

Once control over blood loss and stable normovolemia are gained, specific target hemoglobin levels become more relevant in the decision to transfuse a trauma patient. As for patients in the ICU, there is no consensus around a specific value that can be applied to these patients. However, in the absence of conclusive clinical studies, taking into account the clinical complexity of this group of trauma patients it would seem appropriate to aim for a transfusion trigger of approximately 9-10g/dl hemoglobin.

In hemorraghic shock special concerns regard the extent to which the patient's coagulation system may become exhausted [44]. During massive transfusion

Table 1. Estimated fluid and blood losses based on patient's initial presentation. (Modified from American College of Surgeon Committee on Trauma)

	Class I	Class II	Class III	Class IV
• Blood loss (ml)	<750	750-1500	1500-2000	>2000
• Blood loss (% blood volume)	<15%	15%-30%	30%-40%	>40%
• Pulse rate (beat/min)	<100	>100	>120	>140
• Blood pressure	Normal	Normal	Decreased	Decreased
• Pulse pressure	Normal or increased	Decreased	Decreased	Decreased
• Respiration rate	14-20	20-30	30-40	>40
• Urine output (ml/h)	>30	20-30	5-15	Negligible
• Central nervous system/ mental status	Anxious (slightly)	Anxious (seriously)	Anxious, confused	Confused, lethargic
• Fluid replacement (3:1 rule)	Crystalloid	Crystalloid	Crystalloid + blood	Crystalloid + blood

microvascular bleeding and/or diffuse oozing is often observed. These are partially attributable to a coagulopathy derived from the dilution of platelet and coagulation factors. Since the introduction of pure component therapy, dilutional coagulopathies are more frequently observed in massively transfused patients. The generally accepted rule, although without solid evidence, states that hemostasis is compromised when plasma coagulation factors are decreased to one third of normal [45]. Unfortunately, the activated partial thromboplastin time (APTT) and prothrombin time (PT) are of limited value if used as solitary tests and as an indication for fresh frozen plasma (FFP) supplementation. The abnormal results should not be interpreted without evaluating the clinical picture at the same time. APTT and PT are significantly prolonged at the early stages of blood loss without definite correlation to a bleeding tendency [46]. However, the probability of clinical coagulopathy increases when APTT and PT exceed the normal mean by more than 1.5-fold [47]. When associated with abnormal bleeding these deviations can be used as a signal to use FFP. Moreover, from a practical point of view, the supplementation of FFP should be considered after one blood volume is lost and definitely started before blood loss equals 150% [48].

During massive blood loss the decay of platelets is quite unpredictable and the need for platelet support should be based on repeated platelet counts. The average patient becomes thrombocytopenic after losing two blood volumes but individual variation is great. Accordingly to recently revised guidelines, platelets should be maintained above $50 \cdot 10^9$ during active bleeding. However in patients suffering from multiple high energy trauma, particularly those with central nervous system injuries, values above $100 \cdot 10^9/l$ have been recommended [9].

Moreover, one of the most common causes of coagulopathy in patients receiving massive transfusion for hemorragic shock is hypothermia, as there is a nearly linear relationship between temperature, PT, PTT and platelet function. Coagulopathy due to hypothermia is usually difficult to diagnose because in the majority of patients the coagulation factors, although decreased by dilution, are sufficient for coagulation, and since diagnostic tests are performed in the laboratory at 37°C, their resulting values are within the range of normality. However, in spite of normal laboratory results the majority of patients improperly receive cold FFP to correct bleeding so that the hypothermia-associated coagulopathy is perpetuated.

In some cases microvascular bleeding in patients receiving multiple transfusions for hemorrhagic shock may be caused by disseminated intravascular coagulation (DIC) [49]. The presence of DIC should always be considered as a cause for hemorrhage when severe and extensive tissue trauma occurs, especially when the brain is involved. Indeed massive activation of the hemostatic system induced by trauma may be so powerful that it exceeds the capacity of antithrombin mechanisms to control it, thus precipitating a complex series of reactions leading to systemic activation of the hemostatic system and systemic inflammatory processes. The result of there processes is widespread damage to organs (mainly lungs, kidney, brain and skin) finally causing in a multiple organs deficiency syndrome (MODS).

When a patient is suspected of having DIC or a high risk of DIC, clinical and laboratory examination should be carried out at short intervals. Unfortunately in trauma patients some of the clinical signs of DIC (alteration of mental status, reduced PaO_2 and diuresis,elevated values for serum urea and creatinine) are disguised by those of the traumatic shock itself. Thus in trauma patients the diagnosis should rely on careful observation of the patient's clinical condition evolution and the laboratory hemostatic parameters. Blood samples from patients with suspected DIC should be tested for signs of: increased activation and consumption of platelets (low platelet count), increased activation and consumption of coagulation factors (prolonged APTT and PT, reduced fibrinogen levels, abnormal levels of prothrombin fragment 1,2, fibrinopeptide A, thrombin-antithrombin complexes and soluble fibrin in the plasma), increased activation and consumption of fibrinolysis factors (high D-dimers levels and plasmin-antiplasmin complexes) increased consumption of coagulation inhibition factors (low levels of antithrombin III and protein C and S), increased sequestration of erythrocytes (microangiopathic hemolytic anemia and schistocytes) [50].

Treatment for DIC associated with severe trauma is usually a very difficult task. A detailed discussion on the different therapeutical approaches is well beyond the aims of this chapter, however, it should be kept in mind that the most effective approach is to eliminate the underlying factors that have triggered DIC. Recently, satisfying results in the prevention and treatment of DIC have been reported with the use of large doses of antithrombin concentrates [51, 52].

As can be easily imagined, the alternatives to allogeneic blood transfusion in these patients is very limited. The only currently available strategy is represented by perioperative blood salvage. Beside some anecdotal cases, in which patients survived episodes of massive hemorrhage only with the aid of intraoperative cell salvage [53], the efficacy of this procedure in trauma patients has also been documented in several large studies [53-55]. However its use in open injury is limited as contaminated wounds are generally considered, by most authors, to preclude the use of any cell salvage. Indeed, no existing system of blood filtering or washing can completely eliminate bacteria [56]. Although some reports refer to positive outcome of patients receiving contaminated salvaged blood, the use of blood recovered from a contaminated field is justified only for life-threatening bleeding with no available banked blood [53, 56].

Critical patients

These are usually trauma patients in whom anemia is caused by the traumatic event and who are candidates for a surgical operation that, in some cases, is delayed by a few days. In this group of patients, once normovolemia is gained, a more conservative transfusion practice can be adopted, as the rate of blood loss generally allows the effective activation of adaptation mechanisms (increased cardiac output as a consequence of enhanced preload and increased afterload induced by reduced viscosity and a rightward shift of the hemoglobin-oxygen dissociation curve). Thus under these conditions oxygen delivery is generally adequate in most patients with hemoglobin concentrations above 7 g/dl, assuming that oxygen delivery is not compromised by other physiologic disturbances [9, 10]. However, the decision to administer RBC transfusion should be determined by evaluating the rate of ongoing blood loss and the likelihood of continuing losses, evidence of organ compromise, the patient's age and the risk or presence of cardiovascular or pulmonary disease [57, 58].

Moreover, this category of patients is particularly interesting as far as transfusion treatment is concerned because some form of blood conservation can be applied. In most of the patients undergoing surgical operations, intraoperative and postoperative RBCs salvage can be successfully used. However, as many patients, at the time of the operation, have low hematocrit levels and the volume of RBCs salvaged is minimal, we utilise a "stand-by procedure" that consists of mounting the aspiration set and reservoir, while the washing device is used only if the volume of RBCs collected is considered by the anaesthesiologist to be clinically useful.

Moreover for patients whose surgical procedure is delayed by 3-4 days, an effective alternative to reduce the transfusion of allogeneic blood may be represented by the administration of recombinant human EPO (rHuEPO).

In the last few years different studies have addressed the role of rHuEPO in transfusion medicine [59]. These studies clearly demonstrated the efficacy of rHuEPO treatment in surgical setting as a facilitator of autologous blood donation, thus reducing the risk of allogeneic transfusion in patients scheduled for elective surgery [60-62].

Recently, some studies have also evaluated the role of rHuEPO in those subgroups of patients for whom preoperative autologous blood donation is not feasible. These include patients with anemia or other disorders precluding donation, patients with limited time to surgery, and individuals who are unwilling to participate in an autologous blood donation program because of logistical problems or religous beliefs. A reduced transfusion requirement was evident in these studies [63-65]. Thus rHuEPO could be perioperatively usefully employed as an alternative to predonation. It could be used to stimulate erythropoiesis with the aim of expanding the circulatory red cell mass within a short time period (5-6 days) before surgery in order to allow the patient to tolerate peri- and postoperative blood loss by maintaining hematocrit levels compatible with their clinical condition or it can be used in association with normovolemic hemodilution [66]. Administration of rHuEPO also accelerates regeneration of red cells lost during surgery, with a consequent reduction in the transfusion requirement. The need for predeposit can also be avoided.

A short-term perisurgical treatment was used in a pilot study at our institute. Sixteen patients (including trauma patients) for whom predeposit was contraindicated for various clinical or logistical reasons and who were about to undergo major orthopedic surgery with a predicted transfusion requirement of 2-3 units of blood were enrolled in the study. The protocol involved subcutaneous administration of rHuEPO at a daily dose of 100 IU/kg beginning 4 days before surgery (day -4) up to the second day following surgery (day +2). On the first day of treatment, one 200 IU/kg bolus was also administered intravenously. Intravenous iron saccharate was administered concomitantly at a total dose of 600-1 000 mg, according to baseline iron reserve levels. The treatment produced a 2%-7% increase in hematocrit, with an average increase in circulatory RBC mass of some 100 ml (from 0 to 245) before surgery. Of the 16 patients, 12 did not require allogeneic transfusion, whereas a total of 6 units of blood was transfused in the remaining four patients [67]. Although preliminary, these findings suggest that rHuEPO administration together with IV iron during a pre-operative period of 4-5 days is able to stimulate erythropoiesis significantly, expand the circulatory red cell mass and reduce the transfusion requirement in patients who, for clinical or logistic reasons (cardiovascular surgery and cancer patients), are not able to deposit autologous units prior to elective surgery. Because of the short length of treatment, this protocol could also be offered to a proportion of accident patients about to undergo surgery, when surgery is planned to take place 4-5 days after injury.

The risk of incompatible transfusion in trauma patients

A continuously increasing body of evidence shows that incompatible transfusion due to clerical errors occurs at an unacceptable rate and the risk of a fatal acute hemolytic reaction has been demonstrated to exceed that of HIV transmission [68]. Due to the high emotional situation in the emergency room and trauma center, the risk of human errors in patient or specimen identification may be high. Thus written operative procedures to handle these critical situations must be stated and agreed upon by blood bank staff and personnel involved in the management of these patients. These procedures should be targeted to avoid delay in issuing urgent blood support and to prevent AB0 incompatible transfusion. A useful and safe strategy is to avoid the issue of group specific blood units until the patient AB0 group has been determined on two different blood samples collected at separate times: during this period only group 0 units should be transfused. As far as the Rh type of the issued unit is concerned, the first choice is for Rh-negative units. However, according to the age and gender of the patient, the blood inventory availability and the expected requirement for Rh-negative blood units, it can be decided to issue Rh-positive units for male and postmenopausal female. In Rh-negative females of child bearing age, when Rh-negative blood is not available and transfusion is a life saving procedure, Rh-positive blood can be administered followed by adequate doses of anti-D immunoglobulins. Whenever urgency compels the issue of uncrossmatched units, irregular antibody screening of the patient's serum and a complete crossmatch should be simultaneously performed. If the crossmatch is incompatible, the clinical staff has to be immediately notified so that any adverse reaction can be minimized.

Utmost care must be exercised in identification of the patient for whom blood is ordered or is to be transfused. A variety of different strategies has been used to identify emergency room patients. A popular means of patient identification is the use of a unique trauma alphanumeric hospital identification number. However, recently, increased awareness of the risks of clerical error-related incompatible transfusions led to the introduction of systems specifically designed to avoid such errors. One of these is a mechanical barrier as well as a code based identification system to prevent improper transfusions. This system (Bloodloc Safety System) has been field tested and proven to be effective in preventing mistransfusions [69, 70] and seems to be of value also for use in emergency transfusion.

Conclusions

Transfusion in trauma patients may represent a difficult task as few accepted guideline are presently available. The most important measure is to restore intravascular volume through the administration of crystalloid, under a constant control to avoid hypothermia. RBCs should be transfused to provide O_2 carrying capacity. In case of microvascular bleeding normothermia should be achieved and FFP and platelets concentrates can be administered. In the majority of cases, prophylactic infusion of FFP or platelets and indiscriminate administration of calcium or bicarbonate are contraindicated.

In particular patients, some measures of blood conservation such as intra and post-operative salvage can be utilized alone or in combination with rHuEPO in order to expand the circulating RBC mass before surgery or to accelerate the correction of anemia in the postoperative period.

Utmost care must be exercised to avoid clerical error-related incompatible transfusions; these currently represent the most important cause of transfusion related morbidity and mortality.

References

1. Mezrow CK, Bergstein I, Tartter PI (1992) Postoperative infections following autologous and homologous blood transfusions. Transfusion 32:27-30
2. Triulzi DJ, Vanek K, Ryan DH et al (1992) A clinical and immunologic study of blood transfusion and postoperative bacterial infection in spinal surgery. Transfusion 32:517-524
3. Fernandez MC, Gottlieb M, Menitove JE (1992) Blood transfusion and postoperative infection in orthopedic patients. Transfusion 32:318-22
4. Heiss MM, Mempel W, Jauch KW et al (1993) Beneficial effect of autologous blood transfusion on infectious complications after colorectal cancer surgery. Lancet 342:1328-1333
5. Blumberg N, Heal JM (1994) Effect of transfusion on immune function. Cancer recurrence and infection. Arch Pathol Lab Med 118:371-379
6. Nichols PL, Smith JW, Klein DB et al (1984) Risk of infection after penetrating abdominal trauma. N Engl J Med 311:1065-1070
7. National Institutes of Health Consensus Conference (1988) Perioperative red blood cell transfusion. JAMA 260: 2700-2703
8. American College of Physicians (1992) Practice strategies for elective red blood cell transfusion. Ann Intern Med 116:403-406
9. American Society of Anestesiologists Task Force on Blood Component Therapy (1996) Practice Guidelines for blood component therapy: a report. Anesthesiology 84:732-747
10. Consensus statement on red cell transfusion (1994). Br J Anaesth 73:857-859
11. Goodnough LT, Despotist GJ (1995) Establishing practice guidelines for surgical blood management. Am J Surg 170(Suppl 6A):16-20

12. Development Task Force of the College of American Pathologists (1994) Practice parameters for the use of fresh-frozen plasma, cryoprecipitate, and platelets. Fresh-frozen plasma, cryoprecipitate, and platelets administration practice guidelines. JAMA 271:777-781

13. National Institutes of Health Consensus Conference (1985) Fresh-frozen plasma: indications and risks. JAMA 253:551-553

14. National Institutes of Health Consensus Conference (1987) Platelet transfusion therapy. JAMA 257:1777-1780

15. American College of Surgeons Committee on Trauma (1993) Advanced trauma life support program for physicians; Instructor Manual. American College of Surgeons, Chicago, pp 75-110

16. American College of Surgeons Committee on Trauma (1997) Advanced Trauma Life Support for Doctors, Student Course Manual. American College of Surgeons, Chicago

17. Hebert PC, Wells G, Martin C et al (1995) Red cell transfusion practice in intensive care unit: a systematic evaluation. Blood 86:A857

18. Smoller BR, Kruskall MS (1986) Plebotomy for diagnostic laboratory in adults. N Engl J Med 314:1233-1235

19. Rogiers P, Zhang H, Leeman M et al (1997) Erythropoietin in response is blunted in critically ill patients. Int Care Med 23:159-161

20. Messmer K, Sunder-plassmann L, Klovekorn WP et al (1972) Circulatory significance of hemodilution: rheological changes and limitations. Adv Micocirc 4:1-77

21. Stehling L, Esposito B (1989) An analysis of the appropriateness of intraoperative transfusion. Anesth Analg 68:S1-S278

22. Hébert PC, Schweitzer I, Wells GA et al (1994) A survey of red cell transfusion practices in Canadian critical care pratictioners. Clin Invest Med (Abstract)17:B22

23. Bihari D, Smithies M, Gimson A et al (1987) The effects of vasodilatation with prostacyclin on oxigen delivery and uptake in critically ill patients. N Engl J Med 317:397-403

24. Guticrrez G, Pohil RJ (1986) Oxygen consumption is linearly related to O_2 supply in critically ill patients. J Crit Care 1:45-53

25. Cane RD (1990) Hemoglobin: how much is enough? Crit Care Med 18:1046-1047

26. Shoemaker WC, Appel PL, Kram HB (1992) Role of oxygen debt in the development of organ failure, sepsis, and death in high risk surgical patients. Chest 102:208-215

27. Czer LSC, Shoemaker WC (1980) Myocardial performance in critically ill patients: response to whole blood transfusions as a prognostic measure. Crit Care Med 8:710-715

28. Czer LSC, Shoemaker WC (1987) Optimal hematocrit value in critically ill postoperative patients. Surg Gynecol Obster 147:363-368

29. Bayer WL, Coenen WM, Jenkins DC et al (1980) The use of blood and blood component in 1769 patients undergoing open heart surgery. Ann Thorac Surg 29:117-122

30. Spence RK, Carson JA, Poses R et al (1990) Elective surgery without transfusion: influence of preoperative hemoglobin level and blood loss on mortality. Am J Surg 159:320-324

31. Kawaguchi A, Bergsland J, Subramanian S (1984) Total bloodless open heat surgery in the pediatric age group. Circulation 70:1-30

32. Goodnough LT (1996) Current red blood cell transfusion practice. AACN Clinical Issues 7:212-220

33. Hebert PC, Wells G, Marshall J et al (1995) Transfusion requirement in critiacl care. A pilot study. JAMA 273:1439-1444

34. Yu M, Levy M, Smith P et al (1993) Effect of maximizing oxygen delivery on morbidity and mortality rates in critically ill patients. A prospective randomized controlled study. Crit Care Med 21:830-838

35. Corwin HL, Gettinger A, Rodriguez RM et al (1998) Efficacy of recombinant human erythropoietin in the critically ill patient: a randomized double blind placebo controlled trial. Crit Care Med 26(Suppl 1):A23

36. Lovric V (1984) Alterations in blood components during storage and their clinical significance. Anaesth Intensive Care 12:246-251

37. Marik PE, Sibbad WJ (1993) Effect of stored-blood transfsuion on oxygen delivery in patients with sepsis. JAMA 269:3024-3029

38. Canizaro PC, Shires GT (1973) Fluid resuscitation in severely injured. Surg Clin North Am 53:1341-1366

39. Ferrara A, Mac Arthur JD, Wright HK et al (1990) Hypotermia and acidosis worsen coagulopathy in the patients requiring massive transfusion. Am J Surg 160:515-518

40. Farber JL, Chien KR, Mittnacht Jr (1981) The pathogenesis of irreversible cell injury in ischemia. Am J Pathol 102:271-281

41. Jurkovic GJ, Greiser WB, Luterman A et al (1987) Hypotermia in trauma victims: ominous predictor of survival. J Trauma 27:1019-1024

42. Wildenthal K, Mierzwiak DS, Myers RW et al (1968) Effect of acute lactic acidosis on the left ventricular performance. Am J Physiol 214:1352-1359

43. Benjamin E, Oropello JM, Abalos AM et al (1994) Effects of acid-base correction on hemodynamics, oxygen dynamics, and resuscitability in severe canine hemorrhagic shock. Crit Care Med 22:1616-1623

44. Counts RB, Haisch C, Simon TL et al (1979) Hemostasis in massively transfused patients. Ann Surg 190:91-99

45. Lundsgaard-Hansen P (1992) Treatment of acute blood loss. Vox Sang 2:57-63

46. Leslie SD, Toy PTCY (1991) Laboratory hemostatic abnormalities in massively transfused patients given red cells and crystalloid. Am J Clin Pathol 96:770-773

47. Ciavarella D, Reed RL, Counts RB et al (1987) Clotting factors level and the risk of diffuse microvascular bleeding in the massively transfused patients. Br J Haematol 67:365-368

48. Hippala ST, Myllyla GJ, Vahtera EM (1995) Hemstatic factors and replacement of major blood loss with plasma-poor red cell concentrates. Anesth Analg 81:360-365

49. Bick RL (1994) Disseminated intravascular coagulation. Clin Lab Med 14:729-768

50. Jorgensen M, Gustafsen KB, Ernst S et al (1992) Disseminated intravascular coagulation in critically ill patients. Intensive Care World 9:108-114

51. Albert J, Blomquist H, Gardlund B et al (1992) Effect of antithrombin concentrate on hemostatic variables in critically ill patients. Acta Anaesthesiol Scand 36:745-752

52. Nast-Kolb D, Waydhas C, Jochum M, Schweiberer L (1994) Early antithrombin III treatment of patients with severe multiple injuries. Intens Care Med 20(Suppl 1):121

53. Desmond MJ, Thomas MJG, Gillon Jand Fox MA (1996) Perioperative red cell salvage. Transfusion 36:644-651

54. Giordano GF, Giordano DM, Wallace BA et al (1993) An analysis of 9918 consecutive perioperative autotransfusions. Surg Gynecol Obstet 176:103-110

55. Cavalieri S, Riou B, Roche S et al (1994) Intraoperative autologous transfusion in emergency surgery for spine trauma. J Trauma 36:639-644

56. Dzik WH, Sherburne B (1990) Intraoperative blood salvage: medical controversies. Transf Med Rev IV 3:208-235

57. Expert Working Group (1997) Guidelines for red blood cell and plasma transfusion for adults and children. Can Med Assoc J 156(Suppl 11):1-24

58. Welch HG, Meehan KR, Goodnough LT (1992) Prudent strategies for elective red blood cell transfusion. Ann Int Med 116:393-402

59. Spivak JL (1994) Recombinant human erythropoietin and its role in transfusion medicine. Transfusion 34:1-4
60. Goodnough LT, Rudnick S, Price TH et al (1989) Increased preoperative collection of autologous blood with recombinant human erythropoietin therapy. N Engl J Med 321:1163-1168
61. Mercuriali F, Zanella A, Barosi G et al (1993) Use of erythropoietin to increase the volume of autologous blood donated by orthopedic patients. Transfusion 33:55-60
62. Cazzola M, Mercuriali F, Brugnara C (1997) Use of recombinant human erythropoietin outside the setting of uraemia. Blood 89:4248-4267
63. D'Ambra MN, Lynch KE, Boccagno J, Vlahakes GJ (1992) The effect of perioperative administration of recombinant human erythropoietin (rHuEPO) in CABG patients: a double blind, placebo controlled trial. Anesthesiology 77:A159
64. Canadian Orthopedic Perioperative Erythropoietin Study Group (1993) Effectiveness of perioperative recombinant human erythropoietin in elective hip replacement. Lancet 341:1227-1232
65. Stowell C (1995) Epoetin alfa reduces perioperative transfusion requirements in patients undergoing major orthopedic surgery. Transfusion 35:S27
66. Monk TG, Goodnough LT, Andriole GL et al (1994) Preoperative recombinant human erythropoietin improves outcome with acute normovolemic hemodilution. (Abstract A210) Blood 84 (Supp 1):A64
67. Mercuriali F, Inghilleri G, Biffi E, Colotti MT (1997) Short-term, low dose recombinant human erythropoietin administration in surgery. Br J Anesthesia 78(Suppl 1):64
68. Wenz B, Mercuriali F, AuBuchon JP (1997) Practical methods to improve transfusion safety by using novel blood unit and patient identification systems. AJCP 107(Suppl 1):12-16
69. Mercuriali F, Inghilleri G, Colotti MT et al (1996) Bedside transfusion errors: analysis of 2 years' use of a system to monitor and prevent transfusion errors. Vox Sang 70:16-20
70. Wenz B, Burns ER (1991) Improvement in transfusion safety using a new blood unit and patient identification system as part of safe transfusion practice. Transfusion 31:401-403

Chapter 19

Update on cardiopulmonary resuscitation: guidelines for volunteers

E. Cerchiari, G. Sesana

The response to cardiac arrest has been well standardised and is widely accepted throughout the world as a stepwise response represented by the "chain of survival" [1], in which different actors play different roles according to their level of proficiency and training.

The clinical guidelines have been clearly and universally defined by the ILCOR Advisory Statements – a consensus document approved by all major CPR organisations throughout the world and representing the state of the art reference in CPR, to which the scientific international community should refer to [2].

The teaching and training modalities for each level of proficiency have been defined by the ILCOR-based 1998 European Resuscitation Guidelines, which, promoting the development of a European network of ERC-recognised CPR schools, represent the reference for European countries in terms of CPR teaching and training [3].

In the field of cardiopulmonary resuscitation, volunteers can be defined as individuals not belonging to a health care professional profile who are willing to be trained and to perform CPR if needed. Guidelines for clinical practice and teaching/training modalities are related to the role played within the chain of survival and cannot differ regardless of whether such a role is played by a volunteer or a professional.

Within this scope two major target groups can be identified.

1. Lay people: defined as the first individual to witness an acute emergency event and having a central role in organizing early access and early basic life support (BLS) (one rescuer and without instruments) – the first and second link in the chain of survival. The witness of an out-of-hospital cardiac emergency is more likely to be a non-health care professional, whose probability of witnessing cardiac emergencies in his lifespan is relatively low.

2. Personnel employed on first tier ambulances, who, in our country, have not qualified by enrolling in a national curriculum and who, in some areas, can operate on a volunteer basis. According to the role assigned in other countries to first tier ambulances, such personnel should be prepared to perform early BLS (two rescuer BLS with instruments) and early defibrillation – the second and third links in the chain of survival. The probability of personnel employed in a first tier ambulance responding to a cardiac arrest is high and therefore requires equipment and training based on the best standard of performance.

Role of lay people

The role of lay people in case of unexpected emergency is essential to alert the emergency medical system (EMS), provide reliable information and initiate bystander CPR, the latter being known to correlate with improved outcome following cardiac arrest. CPR is an important lifesaving technique that can be taught to most lay people [4].

For this reason in some areas, initiatives to provide systematic CPR training for lay people have been undertaken; however, this has not led to a satisfactory incidence of bystander CPR [4-6]. Numerous reasons have been identified for the low success rate of traditional CPR training programs in increasing the incidence of bystander CPR:

1. while more than 75% of out-of-hospital cardiac arrests occur at home, the older population most likely to be present is rarely trained in CPR [7];
2. most CPR training is ill-suited for older audiences, because it is classroom-based and taught in the workplace [8];
3. difficulty in skill retention is due to the complexity of the sequence of action and the low relevance of CPR program contents to CPR performance [4-7];
4. there are often problems with instructors' competence [9].

For these reasons, in recent years, all available guidelines for BLS [10-12] have focused on lay people training and have led to the design of simpler medical contents; improved appeal of teaching methodologies; discussion of specific items relevant to lay people, such as reluctance to perform, fear of responsibility and infection; and, finally, removal of formal testing. Even further in the direction of BLS guidelines simplification are the most recent ILCOR Advisory Statements [2] and the ILCOR - based European Resuscitation Council guidelines [3].

The issue of lay people training in BLS has been addressed not only in terms of simplification of contents but also in terms of analysing the teaching/training methodologies in order to try and identify problems with the traditional CPR training methods, when applied to lay people training [5-9, 13-16]:

1. logistic obstacles associated with classroom learning (travel time and inconvenience);
2. psychological barriers and distractions (performance anxiety, unfamiliar setting);
3. mismatch of participants' expectations and actual course content;
4. use of unfamiliar terminology during instruction;
5. delay between instruction of detailed sequence and opportunity for manikin practice;
6. limited time for manikin practice;
7. course content unrelated to performance of CPR;
8. unfocused instruction;
9. lack of meaningful supervision and feedback by instructors.

Therefore, new initiatives for lay people training are under study and have provided encouraging results. For example significant simplification of the sequence of action – reduced from 8-steps to 4-steps – [17] and home mailing of a 34' video self-instruction with inexpensive manikin for a "practice-as you watch" approach achieved better results in skill retention than traditional methods.

It can be concluded that for lay people training BLS guidelines are simple and well-defined, whereas teaching methodologies need to be adjusted , adopting new methodologies and media in order to become appealing and convenient to the different target groups.

Role of volunteer personnel staffing first tier ambulances

The knowledge and skills required for personnel employed on first tier ambulances are the same whether paid or volunteer and is a function of the design of the system, the role assigned within the specific EMS system to the ambulance, and the legislative/curricular national standards.

Throughout the world several EMS models have been developed depending on the country's demographic, cultural and political system; the vast majority, however, are two-tiered systems [19, 20]. Thus, there is a high number of first tier units with personnel qualified at BLS level and therefore, less expensive, widely distributed in order to guarantee a fast response and adequate to satisfy most of the calls. The second tier units, of which there are fewer, are staffed with personnel trained in ALS (advanced life support) treatment; they are therefore more qualified to respond, together with the BLS units, to emergencies requiring a higher level of care. In some rural areas, where second tier response time may be too high, first tier responding units have been upgraded to provide, besides early defibrillation, venous cannulation and airway management [21].

In all systems the tasks required from the first responding units, and, therefore, the equipment required and training of personnel employed, are well defined and represent an international consensus: a BLS team is composed of at least two individuals, better three, all trained to guarantee extrication and immobilization, basic CPR with adjuncts, external hemorrhage control, vital signs assessment, oxygen administration, assisted and positive-pressure ventilation, and on-scene triage. According to the specific system requirements, additional skills have been included, such as airway control and venous cannulation for massive infusion [19, 20].

In terms of CPR, personnel employed on BLS ambulances should be trained to provide, besides one-rescuer CPR (i.e., lay people), two-rescuer CPR in adults and children, with adjuncts for airway control, oxygen administration and ventilation (at different levels of complexity) and maneuvers for management of airway obstruction and semi-automatic defibrillation [2, 3, 10, 11].

Since the chances of successfully resuscitating a ventricular fibrillation decrease by 7%-8% at every minute delay in defibrillation [22-24], there is worldwide agreement that first responding units should all be equipped to provide early semi-automatic defibrillation and that personnel should all be trained in the skill of semi-automatic defibrillation [25-27]. Addition of a defibrillation capability to BLS function has dramatically increased, by a factor of 5, chances of survival after cardiac arrest [1].

In most parts of the world, the personnel staffing BLS ambulances are dedicated professionals with a defined professional profile and a national standard curriculum. These emergency medical technicians (EMTs) have a minimum training level ranging between 120 and 520 h with an average of 150 h [19, 20].

In our country personnel employed for the BLS rescue team do not have a national standard curriculum and, therefore, whether paid or volunteer, do not have homogeneous knowledge and skills. In some areas BLS ambulances are staffed with registered nurses, which is the only health care professional profile in the field of emergency care, besides medical doctors.

With the existing legislation in Italy, defibrillation can be performed by medical doctors and by nurses in the out-of hospital field as long as the procedure follows established protocols and stays and within the scope of a quality control program supervised by the physician in charge of the EMS [28].

State of the art care in out-of-hospital management of cardiac arrest worldwide requires that defibrillation and CPR skills are provided as soon as possible after the acute event. Therefore in order to provide Italian citizens with state of the art EMS care, different levels of interventions are urgently needed:

1. staff all first responding ambulances with a registered nurse in order to be able to implement early defibrillation immediately;
2. define a national curriculum (training program, assessment and periodicity of reassessment) for basic ambulance staff, whether paid or volunteer personnel: the definition of a homogeneous level of knowledge and skills should include the capability of utilizing semi-automatic defibrillation;
3. promote legislation to authorize lay people to perform defibrillation: it has been projected that public access defibrillation can save as much as 30% of lives by anticipation of defibrillation prior to arrival of EMS response [29]. Lay people have been recently reported to be able to effectively perform defibrillation whether trained or not [30];
4. the Italian medical scientific community should take active part in promoting generalized CPR training of the population, legislation allowing public access defibrillation and definition of a national standard curriculum for personnel employed on first and second tier units.

In our country systematic CPR training programs are not being conducted, not even among health professionals. The recent introduction of emergency care in the medical doctor curriculum has not increased CPR skills among young medical graduates [31].

Despite international recognition of the need for periodic CPR re-training for all healthcare professionals, based on the finding that CPR skills decay rapidly [32], that awareness of inadequate performance may not be present [33] and that maintenance of adequate performance improves outcome [34], in Italy requirements of proficiency or competence during professional life are not defined, neither for medical doctors nor for registered nurses.

In our country, since systematic CPR training programs are not being conducted, it is important that all efforts are coordinated towards the common goal of standardising and promoting CPR and that priorities are identified. An effort in this direction has been made by the Italian Resuscitation Council (IRC) with its consensus document on BLS teaching [12] and on early defibrillation. Target pop-

ulations to be trained in BLS are, in decreasing order of priority:
1. personnel, volunteer or paid, employed on EMS ambulances;
2. physicians and nurses, whether employed in hospitals or not;
3. personnel, volunteer or paid, employed in patient transport – non EMS;
4. students of medical and nursing schools;
5. personnel involved in responding to nonmedical emergencies (policemen, firemen, etc.);
6. families of cardiopathic patients, driver education schools, high schools;
7. lay people.

The standardisation of BLS training was promoted by the IRC, which also identified two major target groups and provided an accurate description of training contents, didactic modules, course structures, certification and retraining frequency (Table 1) [12].

Table 1. Levels of basic life support training

Training groups	Category A	Category B
Probability of responding to cardiac arrest	Low Noninstitutional	High Institutional responsibility
Target populations	Lay people Emergency personnel: policemen, firemen General practitioners	EMS ambulance personnel (volunteer or paid) Students of medical and nursing schools Physicians and nurses of health care institutions
Skills	Evaluation Access to EMS One-rescuer CPR Signs of cardiac attack	As category A and: Two rescuer CPR (adults and children) Use of adjuncts for airway, oxigen administration, ventilation, and aspiration Sequence for airway obstruction
Duration	4 h, in two sessions 1 h teaching, 7 h training	8 h, in two sessions 1 h teaching, 7 h training
Course structure	Class size: max 20-30 Training: 1 instructor, 1 manikin, 6 trainees	Class size: max 20-30 Training: 1 instructor, 1 manikin, 6 trainees
Final evaluation	Only for training purposes Not mandatory or formal	Mandatory final test (pass >75%): skill test, multiple choice
Retraining frequency	Volunteer for lay Strongly advised: 2 years	Every 12 months: 2 h retraining, skill test performance
Instructors	Specifically trained Lay people with medical supervision	Specific + standardised training Physicians + nurses
Adjunctive modules	Risk factors (30 min)	Risk factors (30 min) Signs of cardiac attack (30 min)
Highly recommended		Semi-automatic defibrillation (4 h)

Standardisation was achieved also by thorough definition of the training program for instructors', which includes course and supervised instruction together with frequent update meetings and precise definition of requirements to develop a qualified training centre, in order to develop a national network of highly qualified and homogenous training centres.

Obviously, such initiatives are designed with the superior objective of maintaining homogeneity within the country and with other European countries. Therefore, further specifications are needed for adapting to the various national cultures and the internationally approved ILCOR Advisory Statements for clinical practice [2] and the ERC teaching guidelines for different levels of proficiency [3].

References

1. Cummins RO, Ornato JP, Thies WH, Pepe PE (1991) Improving survival from sudden cardiac arrest: the "chain of survival" concept. A statement for health professionals from the Advanced Cardiac Life Support Subcommittee and the Emergency Cardiac Care Committee, American Heart Association. Circulation 83:1832-1847
2. Handley AJ, Becker LB, Allen M, van Drenth A, Kramer EB, Montgomery WH (1997) Basic Life Support Working Group of the International Liaison Committee on Resuscitation – ILCOR. Single rescuer adult basic life Support. Resuscitation 34:101-108
3. Handley AJ, Bahr J, Baskett P, Bossaert L, Chamberlain D, Dick W, Ekstrom L, Juchems R, Kettler D, Marsden A, Moeschler O, Monsieurs K, Parr M, Petit P, Van Drenth A (1998) Working Group on Basic Life Support. The 1998 European Resuscitation Guidelines for Adult Single Rescuer Basic Life Support. Resuscitation 37:67-800
4. Cummins RO, Eisenberg MS (1985) Pre-hospital cardiopulmonary resuscitation. Is it effective? J Am Med Assoc 253:2408-2412
5. Gallagher ED, Lombardi G, Gennis P (1995) Effectiveness of bystander cardiopulmonary resuscitation and survival following out-of hospital cardiac arrest. J Am Med Assoc 274:1922-1925
6. Litwin PE, Eisenberg MS, Hallstrom AP, Cummins RO (1987) The location of collapse and its effect on survival from cardiac arrest. Ann Emerg Med 16:787-791
7. Goldberg JJ, Gore JM, Love DG, Ockene JK, Dalen JE (1984) Layperson CPR – are we training the right people? Ann Emerg Med 13:701-704
8. Brennan RT, Braslow A (1995) Skill mastery in cardiopulmonary resuscitation training classes. Am J Emerg Med 13:505-508
9. Kaye W, Rallis S, Mancini ME et al (1991) The problem of poor retention of cardiopulmonary resuscitation skills may lie with the instructor not the learner or the curriculum. Resuscitation 21:67-87
10. Emergency Cardiac Care Committee and Subcommittees, American Heart Association (1992) Guidelines for cardiopulmonary resuscitation and emergency cardiac care Part II. Adult Basic Life Support. J Am Med Assoc 268:2184-2198
11. Basic Life Support Working Party of the European Resuscitation Council (1992) Guidelines for basic life support. Resuscitation 24:103-110
12. Italian Resuscitation Council (1997) Raccomandazioni per la formazione al basic life support. Minerva Anestesiol 63:93-98
13. Wik L, Brennan RT, Braslow A (1995) A peer training model for instruction of basic life support. Resuscitation 29:119-128

14. Flint LS, Billi JE, Kelley K, Mandel L, Newell L, Stapleton ER (1993) Education in adult basic life support training programs. Ann Emerg Med 22:466-474
15. Weaver FJ, Ramirez AG, Drofman SB, Raizner AE (1979) Trainee's retention of cardiopulmonary resuscitation: how quickly do they forget. J Am Med Assoc 241:901-903
16. Wilson E, Brooks B, Tweed WA (1983) CPR skills retention of lay basic rescuers. Ann Emerg Med 12:482
17. Handley JA, Handley AJ (1998) Four step CPR – improving skill retention. Resuscitation 36:3-8
18. Braslow A, Brennan RT, Newman MM, Bircher NG, Batcheller AM, Kaye W (1997) CPR training without an instructor: development and evaluation of a video self-instructional for effective performance of cardiopulmonary resuscitation. Resuscitation 34:207-220
19. EMS National Association of EMS physicians (1989) In: Kuehl AE (ed) EMS medical director handbook. Mosby, St Louis, pp 39-48
20. Bossaert L(1991) The complexity of comparing different EMS systems: a survey of EMS systems in Europe. Ann Emerg Med 22:99-102
21. Gallaehr JE, Vukov LF (1993) Defining the benefits of rural emergency medical technicians defibrillation. Ann Emerg Med 22:108-112
22. Larsen M, Eisemberg M, Cummins L, Hallstrom A (1993) Predicting survival from out-of-hospital cardiac arrest: a graphic model. Ann Emerg Med 22:1652-1658
23. Weaver WD, Cobb LA, Hallstrom AP et al (1986) Factors influencing survival after out-of-hospital cardiac arrest. J Am Coll Cardiol 7:752-757
24. Weaver WD, Cobb LA Hallstrom AP et al (1986) Considerations for improving survival from out-of-hospital cardiac arrest. Ann Emerg Med 15:1181-1186
25. Advanced Life Support Working Group of the International Liasion Committee on Resuscitation – ILCOR (1997) Early defibrillation. An advisory statement by the Advanced Life Support Working Group of the International Liasion Committee on Resuscitation. Resuscitation 34:113-115
26. Bossaert L, Handley A, Marsden A et al (1998) Early defibrillation. Task force European Resuscitation Council guidelines for the use of automated external defibrillators by EMS providers and first responders. Resuscitation 37:91-94
27. Weisfeldt ML, Kerber RE, Mc Cormick P et al (1995) Public access defibrillation. A statement for the healthcare professionals from the American Heart Association Task force on automatic external defibrillation. Circulation 92:2763
28. Decreto Presidente della Repubblica 27 Marzo 1992
29. Martens P, Calle P, Vanhaute O and the Belgian Cardio Pulmonary Cerebral Resuscitation Study Group (1998) Theoretical calculation of maximum attainable benefit of public access defibrillation in Belgium. Resuscitation 36:161-163
30. Fromm RE, Varon J (1997) Automated external versus blind manual defibrillation by untrained lay rescuers. Resuscitation 33:219-221
31. Parise G, Palmussi G, Laganà D et al (1994) Neolaureato e nozioni di pronto soccorso: indagine conoscitiva su un campione di 1497 medici. Federazione Medica 20:318-319
32. Weaver FJ, Ramirez AG, Dorman SB et al (1979) Trainees retention of cardiopulmonary resuscitation: how quickly do they forget? J Am Med Assoc 241:901-903
33. KuhnigK H, Sefrin P, Paulus TH (1994) Skills and self-assessment in cardiopulmonary resuscitation of the hospital nursing staff. Eur J Emerg Med 1:193-198
34. Bernard WN, Tundorf H, Cotrell JE et al (1979) Impact of cardiopulmonary resuscitation training on resuscitation. Crit Care Med 22:741-749

Chapter 20

Guidelines on trauma management

A.J. Sutcliffe

Traditional medical practice is based on knowledge of current research, experience and common sense, all of which are variables specific to an individual. Thus, there is a tendency for each doctor to manage the same condition slightly differently. Usually, patients recover well. Because some differences in clinical management may have an impact on cost-effective use of finite resources, doctors are being asked to justify their practice.

Managed care and evidence-based medicine have been advocated, usually by governments or insurance companies. Doctors are suspicious of these initiatives fearing that they are an attempt to limit clinical freedom and control costs. Consequently, the medical profession has not wholeheartedly accepted the concept of evidence-based medicine [1]. Nevertheless, some Trauma Centres have accepted the challenge and are attempting to improve the cost-effectiveness of their services by methods which do not prohibit any treatment options. A beneficial effect has been demonstrated from co-ordinated patient care and improved awareness of the resources that specific clinical practices consume [2].

Evidence-based medicine can be a useful tool for enabling doctors to keep abreast of current knowledge, enhancing their critical appraisal skills and helping them to decide the most appropriate and effective treatment for their patients [3]. For trauma care, there is a dearth of good quality scientific evidence to prove that current treatments have a positive effect on outcome [4]. Despite this, many standards, protocols, guidelines and recommendations have been developed and implemented.

Standards, guidelines and protocols

Standards reflect a high degree of clinical certainty and are intended to be rigidly applied [5, 6]. Sterile technique in the operating room is an example. Standards are usually supported by Class 1 evidence. The precise definition of Class 1 evidence varies but is generally considered to comprise data from well designed prospective, randomised, controlled trials [5].

Guidelines are supported by Class 2 evidence obtained from observational, cohort and prevalence studies. Because the supporting evidence provides a lesser degree of clinical certainty, guidelines are more general, less rigid, and convey a philosophy that they should be followed in most cases but are open to individual interpretation. Words such as "may be indicated" are used [6]. Doctors may deviate from the treatment recommended when they believe it is clinically indicated but it is usually wise to record why this was done. The American College of Surgeons (ACS) developed an Advanced Trauma Life Support (ATLS) course in 1989. The course manual [7] and teaching techniques were didactic. Since the course's introduction, it has been changed in the light of new evidence and has become the world wide standard for trauma resuscitation. Strictly, much of the course content should be classified as a guidelines rather than standards. It is clear from the introduction to the manual that this is what the authors intended, because they note that although one method of performing each technique is recommended, there are other acceptable practices.

Protocols, like standards, are explicit in their instructions to the practitioner. They tend to be restricted to a clearly defined group of patients and a single component of treatment. An example is an insulin regime designed to control blood sugar within a specified range.

Standards, protocols and guidelines share several common attributes which are believed to enhance their effectiveness. As far as the evidence permits, they need to be explicit and unambiguous, valid, clinically relevant, appropriate for most clinical needs, accepted by users and easily reviewed and modified in the light of clinical experience and new knowledge [6]. This chapter considers ATLS guidelines for resuscitation and Brain Trauma Foundation (BTF) guidelines for the management of head injury and assesses them in the context of their attributes as described above.

Is the implementation of ATLS guidelines effective in improving outcome?

ATLS guidelines are accepted by most doctors as unambiguous, clinically relevant and appropriate for most trauma patients. Their particular advantage is that all doctors trained in the method will be approaching an individual patient's management from the same knowledge and skill base and will thus be able to work effectively together as a team. Despite the widespread use of ATLS guidelines in hospital, their use outside hospital is less frequent. The absence of pre-hospital ATLS is associated with a deterioration in the condition of trauma patients prior to admission to hospital [8]. Pre-hospital ATLS reduces mortality, disability and hospital length of stay [9]. The improvement in outcome is thought to be due to better airway control, more frequent administration of oxygen, improved spinal immobilisation and better haemorrhage control [10]. ATLS training improves the number of key treatment objectives achieved in the hospital management of simulated trauma patients [11]. These reports support the validity of ATLS guidelines for improving outcome. Therefore, it is disappointing that there continue to be reports of hospital preventable deaths caused by airway compromise and inadequate or delayed fluid resuscitation [12, 13].

Clearly, there is still room for improvement. It is important to clarify why preventable deaths occur. In Canada, patients taken directly to a trauma centre have a better survival rate than those transferred from another hospital [14]. It is suggested that patients are managed less well outside the trauma centre and that improved transport protocols are needed. In the UK, junior doctors are primarily responsible for the reception of severely injured patients but many are unable to attend ATLS training courses because financial support and places in courses are taken up by more senior doctors [15]. An Australian study has suggested that although the medical skills taught in ATLS courses are well applied, team leaders are poor communicators [16]. Communication is not a skill currently incorporated in ATLS training because the guidelines were originally developed for the single-handed doctor. These examples illustrate the value of reviewing the consequences of introducing guidelines. Although guidelines may be inherently useful, their benefits will not be fully realised unless there is guidance on all aspects of care, good communication within the team and appropriate training of team members.

Are ATLS guidelines appropriate for the care of all injured patients?

Because Class 1 evidence is lacking, many ATLS guidelines are based on Class 2 evidence plus the considerable clinical experience of the authors. A report from the ACS challenges some commonly held beliefs about factors predicting adverse outcome. The ACS has chosen to study nine trauma quality indicators. Contrary to expectation, four of these indicators do not appear to predict adverse outcome. These are coma without intubation, laparatomy performed greater than 2 h after injury, time to completion of transfer of greater than 6 h and admission to a nonsurgical service [17]. The reasons for the predictive failure of these indicators are complex.

The first part of ATLS is the primary survey in which the patient is briefly examined and life threatening airway, breathing and circulation abnormalities are identified and treated. The ACS identifies coma without intubation as an indicator which fails to predict an adverse outcome. This may be because in many institutions, emergency room endotracheal intubation is performed by non-anaesthetists and a significant number of mishaps have occurred [18]. In the UK, blind nasal intubation, as advocated in early ATLS courses, is poorly performed by non-anaesthetic personnel [19]. Thus, the theoretical basis for the guidelines is probably valid and the importance of appropriate training and experience is reinforced.

Delay in transfer to the operating room and an associated reduction in blood pressure is reported as a potential cause of preventable death [20] but was not confirmed as a predictive quality indicator by the ACS. In contrast, a landmark paper [21] suggests that in an urban hospital with immediately available skilled surgeons, patients with life threatening haemorrhage from penetrating trauma to the torso do better if fluid resuscitation is delayed until the patient is in the operating room and the bleeding has been surgically controlled. A study from the UK supports this view [22]. It appears that ATLS guidelines relating to rapid restoration of blood pressure are too general and may be inappropriate for some subsets of patients which have yet to be clearly defined.

Furthermore, ATLS guidelines are restricted to the resuscitation period prior to the patient's prompt transfer to theatre for surgery. It is reasonable to suppose that the conduct of surgery and anaesthesia influences outcome independent of the quality of resuscitation. Current practice assumes that all surgical procedures should be definitive but this is no longer certain. Some authors are developing guidelines for damage control surgery, which always involves more than one operative procedure [23-25]. The first operation is restricted to control of life-threatening haemorrhage after which the patient is nursed in intensive care until physiological stability has been restored. Only then, is the patient moved back to the operating room so that definitive surgery can be performed. The philosphy behind damage control surgery is that the severity and duration of profound physiological derangement should be reduced to a minimum in order to reduce the incidence of complications and their associated mortality.

Many of the studies quoted in this and the preceding section use mortality as an outcome measure. Mortality is easy to define; but it is a crude, often insensitive measure of outcome which may be influenced by the implementation of changes in practice advocated by one or more sets of guidelines.

Are ATLS guidelines explicit and unambiguous?

Almost every published paper and chapter about ATLS stresses the need for prompt, accurate resuscitation but few state precisely what the end-points of resuscitation should be. A consensus has yet to be achieved probably because of the lack of appropriate research data. Our inability to initiate appropriate monitoring during the life-saving phase of resuscitation [26] is another limiting factor. In the early phase of resuscitation, we rely on insensitive, intermittent indicators of tissue oxygenation such as pulse rate, blood pressure and urine output. Invasive measures of cardiac output and global tissue oxygenation are only used when the patient has stabilised sufficiently to allow the insertion of complex monitoring devices. Recently, non-invasive techniques for the continuous measurement of cardiopulmonary function and tissue perfusion have been described and may find a place in the emergency room and outside hospital [27]. Even if these non-invasive techniques are adopted widely, it is suggested that computerised analysis of the data may be needed to help the clinician interpret the physiological changes and to decide the most appropriate clinical interventions [26].

A number of rapid infusor systems (RIS) are available which allow the administration of fluid at a rate equal to or greater than the rate of haemorrhage. A recent paper suggests that patients with blood loss exceeding 6l have a greater mortality when treated with a RIS than those who are not [28]. There has been a vociferous response. The authors acknowledge that their study has design flaws [29] but stress that all they wish to do is draw attention to the fact that over as well as under resuscitation may have an adverse effect on outcome. Given that stress has always been placed on giving fluid rapidly and the optimal end-points of resuscitation have not been clearly established, their findings should not be surprising. Their work confirms that evidence for optimal clinical practice is not yet available for the trauma population.

Still more contentious is the issue of which fluid should be used. ATLS guidelines reflect the North American perspective and suggest that crystalloid fluids, then strictly limited amounts of colloid followed by blood should be given. Many other countries have developed guidelines which allow more liberal use of colloids, particularly albumin, but again, blood is recommended to replace blood loss. While all agree that blood should be given in volumes adequate to replace blood loss, the debate about the best fluid to use while blood is cross matched continues. There is no doubt that transfusion practice differs widely between institutions. A systematic review of trials comparing albumin regimes with crystalloid regimes in surgical, trauma and burns patients strongly suggests an increase in mortality when albumin is used in preference to crystalloid [30]. Given the evidence in favour of using crystalloid solutions, this may be an example of a situation in which cost is an appropriate consideration when choosing a therapeutic intervention.

Management of head injury

Management practices for head injury are variable, even in recognised neurosurgical centres [31, 32]. The BTF has issued a document describing the medical management of head injury [5]. For almost all the treatments examined, guidelines are given because there is insufficient evidence to set standards. An example is the guideline which suggests that a minimum systolic blood pressure of 90 mm Hg is required to prevent secondary brain injury. Another more recent retrospective population study indicates that that even transient falls of systolic blood pressure to below 100 mm Hg are associated with a poor outcome particularly for the subset of patients whose initial head injury was relatively minor [33]. This is just one example of the importance of reviewing guidelines regularly and amending them in the light of new evidence. The role of lobectomy for controlling raised intra-cranial pressure is not considered in the BTF guidelines which concentrate on medical interventions. Recent research suggests that for a subset of head injured patients, namely young people with an initial high Glasgow Coma Score (GCS) who subsequently develop high intracranial pressure which is uncontrollable using medical treatments, lobectomy may reduce mortality without increasing the number surviving in a vegetative state [34]. In the future, BTF guidelines may also need amending because there is new evidence that outcome is influenced by different associated factors depending on the severity of head injury [35]. Injury severity score (ISS) influences outcome in patients with an emergency room GCS of between 4 and 12 and age influences outcome when the GCS is 13 or greater. It is important that these factors be taken into consideration when studies comparing different treatments are being used to support evidence-based practice.

Conclusions

Evidence-based guidelines are helpful in promoting improved trauma management but they require continual review and updating. They are ineffective if staff do not have the appropriate training or experience for correct implementation. There is a pressing need for research which provides answers to questions for which there is no convincing evidence [4]. In the future, trauma guidelines may be refined and applied to specific subsets of patients with more specific treatment goals. Better outcome indicators will be identified. Morbidity may prove to be a better discriminator between treatments and replace mortality as an outcome indicator. Patients rather than doctors may prefer quality of life indicators but these are difficult to define and quantify and are rarely used by the medical profession as evidence for guidelines [36].

References

1. Goodman NW (1998) Anaesthesia and evidence based medicine. Anaesth 53:353-368
2. Imami ER, Clevenger FW, Lampard SD et al (1997) Through out analysis of trauma resuscitations with financial impact. J Trauma 42:294-298
3. Cook D (1998) Evidence-based critical care medicine: a potential tool for change. New Horiz 6:20-25
4. Dick WF (1996) Setting standards and implementing quality improvement in trauma care. Eur J Em Med 3:270-273
5. Bullock R, Chesnut RM, Clifton G et al (1995) Guidelines for the management of severe head injury. Brain Trauma Foundation
6. Clemmer TP, Spuhler VJ (1998) Developing and gaining acceptance for patient care protocols. New Horiz 6:12-19
7. Committee on Trauma of the American College of Surgeons (1989) Advanced trauma life support course student manual. American College of Surgeons, Chicago
8. Hu SC, Kao WF (1996) Outcomes in severely ill patients transported without prehospital ALS. Am J Em Med 14:96-88
9. Ali J, Adan RU, Gana TJ et al (1997) Trauma patient outcome after the prehospital trauma life support program. J Trauma 42:1018-1021
10. Ali J, Adan RU, Gana TJ et al (1997) Effect of prehospital trauma life support program on prehospital trauma care. J Trauma 42:786-790
11. Williams MJ, Lockey AS, Culshaw MC (1997) Improved trauma management with advanced trauma life support (ATLS) training. J Accid Emerg Med 14:81-83
12. McDermott FT, Cordner SM, Tremayne AB (1996) Evaluation of the medical management and preventability of death in 137 road traffic fatalities in Victoria, Australia: an overview. J Trauma 40:520-533
13. Arreola-Risa C, Mock CN, Padilla D et al (1995) Trauma care systems in Latin America: the priorities should be prehospital and emergency room management. J Trauma 39:457-462
14. Sampalis JS, Denis R, Frechette P et al (1997) Direct transport to tertiary trauma centers versus transfer from lower level facilities: impact on mortality and morbidity among patients with major trauma. J Trauma 43:288-295
15. Price A, Hughes G (1998) Training in advanced trauma life support. Br Med J 316:878

16. Sugrue M, Seger M, Kerridge R et al (1995) A prospective study of the performance of the trauma team leader. J Trauma 38:79-82

17. Nayduch D, Moylan J, Snyder BL et al (1994) American College of Surgeons trauma quality indicators: an analysis of outcome in a statewide trauma registry. J Trauma 37:565-573

18. Nayyar P, Lisbon A (1997) Non-operating room emergency airway management of endotracheal intubation practices: a survey of anesthesiology program directors. Anesth Analg 85:62-68

19. McHale SP, Brydon CW, Wood ML et al (1994) A survey of nasotracheal intubating skills among Advanced Trauma Life Support course graduates. Br J Anaesth 72:195-197

20. Hoyt DB, Bulger EM, Knudson MM et al (1994) Death in the operating room: an analysis of a multi-center experience. J Trauma 37:426-432

21. Bickell WH, Wall MJ, Pepe PE et al (1994) Immediate versus delayed fluid resuscitation for hypotensive patients with penetrating torso injuries. New Eng J Med 331:1105-1109

22. Shah N, Palmer C, Sharma P (1998) Outcome of raising blood pressure in patients with penetrating trunk wounds. Lancet 351:648-649

23. Rotondo MF, Zonies BA (1997) The damage control sequence and underlying logic. Surg Clin N Am 77(4):761-777

24. Martin RR, Byrne M (1997) Postoperative care and complications of damage control surgery. Surg Clin N Am 77(4):929-942

25. Pourmoghadam KK, Fogler RJ, Shaftan GW (1997) Ligation: an alternative for control of exsanguination in major vascular injuries. J Trauma 43:126-130

26. Shoemaker WC, Peitzman AB, Bellamy R et al (1996) Resuscitation from severe hemorrhage. Crit Care Med 24:512-523

27. Asensio JA, Demetriades D, Berne TV et al (1996) Invasive and noninvasive monitoring for early recognition and treatment of shock in high-risk trauma and surgical patients. Surg Clin N Am 76(4):985-997

28. Hambly PR, Dutton RP (1996) Excess mortality associated with the use of a rapid infusion system at a Level 1 trauma centre. Resuscitation31:127-133

29. Dutton RP (1997) Response to letters. Trauma Care 7:61

30. Cochrane injuries Group Albumin Reviewers (1998) Human albumin administration in critically ill patients: systematic review of randomised controlled trials. Br Med J 317:235-240

31. Ghajar J, Hariri RJ, Narayan RK et al (1995) Survey of critical care management of comatose, head-injured patients in the United States. Crit Care Med 23:560-567

32. Matta B, Menon D (1996) Severe head injury in the United Kingdom and Ireland: a survey of practice and implications for management. Crit Care Med 24:1743-1748

33. Winchell RJ, Simons RK, Hoyt DB (1996) Transient systolic hypotension. A serious problem in the management of head injury. Arch Surg 131:533-539

34. Litofsky NS, Chin LS, Tang G et al (1994) The use of lobectomy in the management of closed-head trauma. Neurosurg 34:628-633

35. Hill DA, Delaney LM, Roncal S (1997) A chi-square automatic interaction detection analysis of factors determining trauma outcomes. J Trauma 42:62-66

36. Grotz M, Hohensee A, Remmers D et al (1997) Rehabilitation results of patients with multiple injuries and multiple organ failure and long-term intensive care. J Trauma 42:919-926

Main symbols

ACS	American College of Surgeons
AG	Anion Gap
AIS	Abbreviated Injury Scale
ALS	Advanced Life Support
APACHE	Acute Physiology and Chronic Health Evaluation
APTT	Activated Partial Thromboplastin Time
ARDS	Adult Respiratory Distress Syndrome
ASCOT	Severity Characterization of Trauma
ATLS	Advanced Trauma Life Support
BAC	Blood Alcohol Concentrations
BE	Base Excess
BTF	Brain Trauma Foundation
CAT	Comprehensive Approach to Trauma
CNS	Central Nervous System
CO	Cardiac Output
COP	Colloid Oncotic Pressure
COPA	Cuffed Oropharyngeal Airway
CPAP	Continuous Positive Airway Pressure
CPK	Creatine Phosphokinase
CPR	Cardiopulmonary Resuscitation
CVP	Central Venous Pressure
DIC	Disseminated Intravascular Coagulation
DRK	Deutsche Red Cross
ELAM-1	Endothelial Leukocyte Adhesion Molecule
EMS	Emergency Medical System
EPO	Erythropoietin
FFP	Fresh Frozen Plasma
FRC	Functional Residual Capacity
GALT	Gut-associated Lymphatic Tissue
GCS	Glasgow Coma Scale
GFR	Glomerular Filtration Rate
GMP-140	Granule Membrane Protein 140
HEMS	Helicopter Emergency Medical System
HES	Hydroxyethyl Starches
HFPV	High Frequency Percussive Ventilation
HR	Heart Rate
HS	Haemorrhagic Shock
ICAM-1	Intercellular Adhesion Molecule-1
ICP	Intracranial Pressure
ICU	Intensive Care Unit
IGSF	Immunoglobulin Superfamily
ISS	Injury Severity Score
ITACCS	International Trauma Anaesthesia and Critical Care Society

LECAM	Leukocyte Endothelial Cell Adhesion Molecule
LFA-1	Lymphocyte Function-Associated Antigen
LMA	Laryngeal Mask Airway
LMA-FT	LMA Fastrach
LSD	Lysergic Acid Diethylamide
LVAS	Linear Visual Analog Score
MAC	Minimum Anaesthetic Concentration
MAP	Mean Arterial Pressure
MDMA	Methylenedioxymethamphetamine
MEGX	Monoethylglycinexylidide
MH	Malignant Hyperpyrexia
MODS	Multiple Organ Dysfunction Syndrome
MOF	Multiple Organ Failure
MPM	Mortality Prediction Models
MTOS	Major Trauma Outcome Study
NO	Nitric Oxide
PACU	Postanaesthesia Care Unit
PAOP	Pulmonary Artery Occlusive Pressure
PCP	Phencyclidine
PCWP	Pulmonary Capillary Wedge Pressure
pHi	Gastric Mucosal pH
PMNs	Polymorphonuclear cells
PS	Probability of Survival
PT	Prothrombin Time
PVR	Pulmonary Vascular Resistances
RAS	Renin-Angiotensin System
RCC	Rescue Coordination Center
rHuEPO	Recombinant Human EPO
RIS	Rapid Infusor Systems
RTS	Revised Trauma Score
RVEDV	Right Ventricular End-Diastolic Volume
SAMU	Service d'Aide Medicale Urgente
SAPS II	Simplified Acute Physiological Score
SAR	Search and Rescue
SIRS	Systemic Inflammatory Response Syndrome
THC	Tetrahydrocannabinol
TRISS	Trauma Score and Injury Severity Score
TS	Trauma Score
TTJV	Transtracheal Jet Ventilation
VCAM-1	Vascular Cell Adhesion Molecule-1
VO_2	Oxygen Consumption
XO	Xanthine Oxidase

Subject index

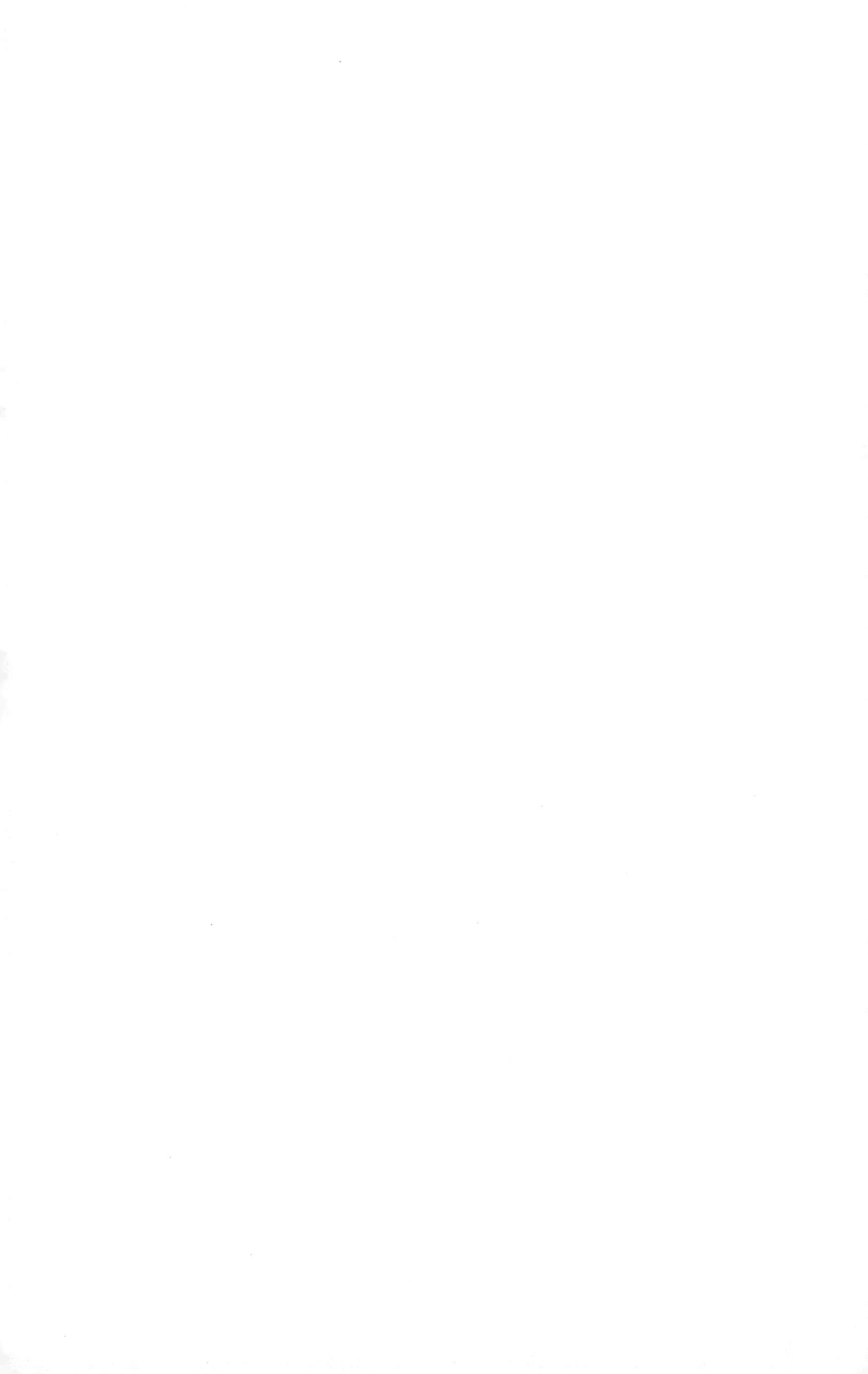

Made in the USA
Monee, IL
07 July 2026